Hydrogen For Health

A Science-Based Guide to
Molecular Hydrogen for
Inflammation, Energy, and Cognitive Health

By John Iovine

Copyright

All Rights Reserved. No part of this book may be reproduced in any manner without written permission from the publisher. While every precaution has been taken in the preparation of this book, the author, the publisher, or the seller assumes no responsibility for errors or omissions. No liability is assumed for damages resulting from the use or misuse of the information contained herein.

READ THIS FIRST – DISCLAIMER
The author has narrated his research experiences in this book by observing and evaluating facts and figures. The reliance on information has been made in good faith and is believed to be reliable, according to the author's best knowledge. The sources of referenced information could change or be updated in the future. The author cannot guarantee the validity and accuracy of the sources, which may change, be modified, updated, or removed in the future, and thus, disclaims himself from any such changes, modifications, updates, and removals. (10)

ISBN: 978-1-62385-031-9 Print
ISBN: 978-1-62385-030-2 eBook

Table of Contents

Introduction 1
   Why This Book Exists — and How to Use It 1
Chapter 1 - What is Hydrogen? 5
Chapter 2 – H2's Unexpected Role in Biology 9
   The Significance of Hydrogen in Medicine 9
Chapter 3 - The Benefits of Hydrogen Therapy 11
   Understanding the Benefits of Hydrogen Gas Therapy 11
Chapter 4 - Maximize Your Experience 15
   Using This Book 15
Chapter 5 - Is Hydrogen Gas Therapy Safe? 19
   FDA Ruling on Hydrogen Safety 20
Chapter 6 - Hydrogen Wellness for Seniors 21
   Improved Cognitive Function 21
Chapter 7 - Hydrogen for Athletes 31
   Athletic Advantages 31
Chapter 8 - Anti-Aging 35
   Anti-Aging Attributes 35
Chapter 9 - Hydrogen For Chronic Illness 37
   Hydrogen's Potential in Diabetes Management 37
Chapter 10 – Hydrogen For Eye Health 45
   How Can Hydrogen Gas Help the Eyes? 46
   Corneal Injuries and Surgery: 51
Chapter 11 - Hydrogen Administration 59
   Incorporating Hydrogen Gas Into a Health Regime 59
Chapter 12 - Hydrogen Generator Products 67
   Hydrogen-Rich Baths and Topical Applications 67
   Water Ionizers (electrolysis machines) 71
Chapter 13 – Conclusions 79
Glossary of Key Terms 81

Introduction

Why This Book Exists — and How to Use It

If you are reading this book, you may be dealing with inflammation that never fully resolves, fatigue that lingers despite good habits, or a sense that your health is slowly slipping, even though you are doing everything you were told to do.

Hydrogen therapy often appears at this stage of the journey.

Is there something small, overlooked, and biologically meaningful that could make a difference?

This book exists to answer that question honestly.

What This Book Is — and Is Not

This is **not** a book about wellness trends, biohacking hype, or dramatic overnight results. It is also **not** a book that asks you to believe anything on faith.

This book examines **molecular hydrogen (H_2)** as a therapeutic agent, *drawing on published research, biological mechanisms, and practical measurement methods,* while clearly stating limitations, uncertainties, and realistic expectations.

If you are looking for *health* guarantees, this book will disappoint you. If you are looking for understanding, it will not.

Why Hydrogen Is Worth Examining at All

Hydrogen is the smallest molecule in the universe. For decades, it was assumed to be biologically inert. That assumption was overturned in 2007, when research demonstrated that molecular hydrogen could selectively reduce harmful oxidative stress in living tissue without disrupting beneficial biological signaling.

Since then, hydrogen has been studied in relation to:
- Oxidative stress and chronic inflammation
- Mitochondrial function and energy production
- Cognitive decline and neurodegenerative disease
- Metabolic dysfunction and insulin resistance
- Recovery from intense physical stress
- Aging-related cellular damage

Importantly, the effects reported in the literature are **modest, measurable, and cumulative**—not dramatic or immediate.

That distinction matters.

A Critical Expectation Reset

One of the most important points in this book is also the easiest to misunderstand:

Hydrogen therapy does not make you "feel" something right away.

Unlike stimulants, painkillers, or hormones, hydrogen's effects are subtle and biological. In most cases, they require instruments—not sensations—to detect.

This book repeatedly emphasizes that point because misunderstanding it leads people to dismiss hydrogen prematurely or exaggerate its effects unrealistically.

Think of hydrogen less like caffeine and more like micronutrients:
- You do not feel them working
- But long-term deficiency or support matters

Who Will Benefit Most From This Book

This book is written for readers who value:

- Evidence over anecdotes
- Measurement over marketing
- Biological plausibility over hype
- Incremental improvement over dramatic promises

You may find this book especially useful if you are:

- Over 40 and noticing slow, systemic decline
- Managing metabolic or inflammatory conditions
- Concerned about cognitive health or aging
- An athlete or active adult focused on recovery
- Skeptical, but curious

How to Read This Book

This book favors caution over enthusiasm and clarity over persuasion. This book is structured to move from **foundational understanding** to **practical application**:

1. What hydrogen is and why it matters biologically
2. What research actually shows—and what it does not
3. Where hydrogen may provide benefit
4. How hydrogen is administered, measured, and evaluated
5. Safety considerations and realistic dosing
6. Practical guidance without exaggeration

You do not need to believe in hydrogen therapy to benefit from this book. You only need to be willing to evaluate evidence carefully.

A Final Clarification Before We Begin

Hydrogen therapy is not a replacement for medical treatment.
It is best viewed as a **complementary, low-risk intervention** that may offer small but meaningful benefits over time.

If hydrogen provides even a 1–2% improvement in biological resilience over the long term, that improvement compounds.

That is the frame this book uses.
Nothing more—and nothing less.

With expectations set correctly, we can begin.

Chapter 1 - What is Hydrogen?

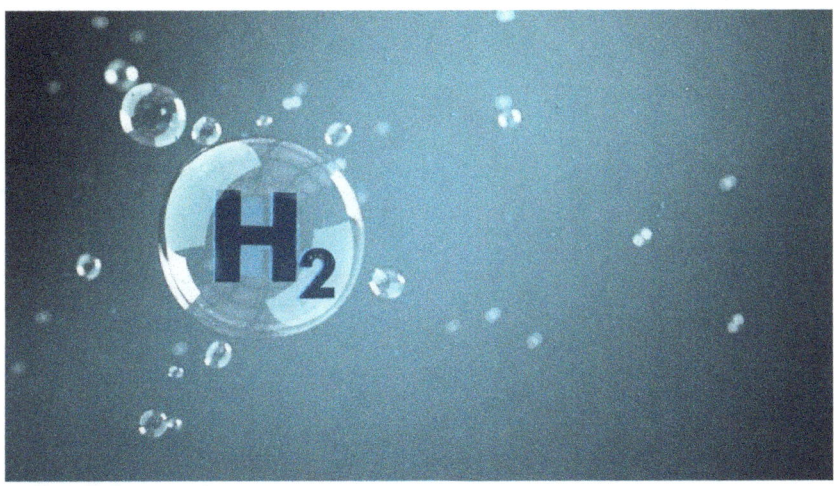

Hydrogen is the most abundant element in the known universe, accounting for most of the mass, except for "Dark Matter." Dark matter is an unidentified mass required in astrophysics to balance the observable phenomena in the universe.

In recent years, the scientific community has reported on the potential hydrogen has for healing and promoting optimal health.

History of Hydrogen

The artificial production of hydrogen gas was first observed in the early 1500s when acids were mixed with metals. In 1671, Robert Boyle recorded the reaction between iron particles and diluted acids, which yields hydrogen.

It wasn't until Henry Cavendish's research during 1766-1781 that it was determined that hydrogen is a separate entity and creates water when burned - the meaning behind the Greek name "hydrogen", which translates to "water-former." The famous combination of Hydrogen (H_2) and oxygen to form water (H_2O).

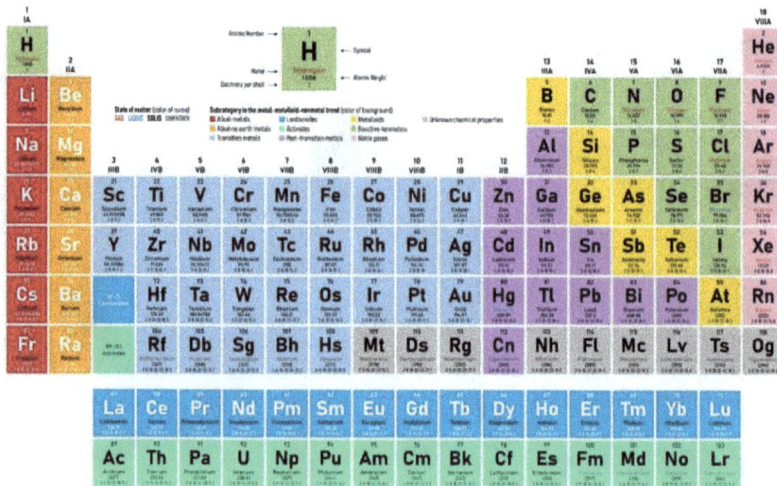

At standard temperature and pressure, hydrogen exists as a colorless, odorless, tasteless gas. It is the lightest element on the periodic table, consisting of a single proton and a single electron.

Its chemical symbol is **H**.

Hydrogen as an Element

Because single hydrogen atoms are highly reactive, they rarely exist independently. Instead, hydrogen naturally bonds with other atoms, or with itself.

When two hydrogen atoms bond, they form molecular hydrogen, written H_2.

This distinction matters.

Throughout this book, the term *hydrogen* refers specifically to **molecular hydrogen (H_2)**, not atomic hydrogen, and not hydrogen bound into other compounds.

A molecule of hydrogen, H2, has an atomic weight of 2.016.

Where We Go Next

The next chapter examines how a molecule long assumed to be biologically inert came to challenge that assumption—and why that shift mattered.

Chapter 2 – H2's Unexpected Role in Biology

The therapeutic potential of hydrogen was unexpected. Without a catalyst, H2 does not react with biological tissues or compounds.

US Naval Divers, when performing deep underwater diving operations, switched from compressed air and breathed a blend of oxygen and hydrogen. This mixed gas combination was chosen because hydrogen is considerably less toxic than nitrogen under pressure in the human body.

Individuals breathing compressed air at great depths can experience "Nitrogen Narcosis," a condition resulting from excessive nitrogen gas accumulation in the blood and muscles. This saturation impairs a diver's cognitive and motor functions, akin to consuming excessive alcohol. Furthermore, a rapid ascent can cause nitrogen gas to bubble out from the blood and muscles, like the bubbling fizz when opening a carbonated drink, leading to a dangerous condition known as decompression sickness or "the bends."

Using hydrogen gas as a component in diving mixtures effectively reduces these deep-diving challenges and continues to do so.

This idea that hydrogen was biologically inert was overthrown in 2007.

The Significance of Hydrogen in Medicine

In 2007, scientists led by Ohsawa discovered that hydrogen gas could notably reduce brain damage in rats that had experienced a type of stroke. In their study, the team caused a stroke by blocking a major artery in the rats' brains and then exposed some of the rats to a chamber filled with 2-4% hydrogen gas. The results showed that the rats that breathed in hydrogen had much less brain damage than those that did not. The researchers suggest that hydrogen works by targeting and neutralizing harmful molecules that can damage cells, although it's more effective against some than others.

Source: I. Ohsawa, M. Ishikawa, K. Takahashi et al., "Hydrogen acts as a therapeutic antioxidant by selectively reducing cytotoxic oxygen radicals," Nature Medicine, vol. 13, no. 6, pp. 688–694, 2007.

Hydrogen gas and hydrogen-infused water have recently gained attention for their potential health benefits, building on more than a decade of research in biological systems. Seniors, often characterized by weakened immune systems, decreased bone density, and reduced cognitive function, may especially benefit from hydrogen therapies. As the smallest molecule, hydrogen can easily penetrate cells, neutralizing harmful free radicals, thus reducing oxidative stress and inflammation.

https://www.hindawi.com/journals/omcl/2012/353152/#B6

Japan's Ministry of Health approved the inhalation of hydrogen gas as advanced medical care for patients with post-cardiac arrest syndrome (PCAS) in November 2016. This treatment quickly sends hydrogen throughout the body, which helps to fight the harmful effects of sudden and severe oxidative stress.

Moreover, Japanese health authorities have also endorsed the use of hydrogen-enriched saline drips to help patients recover from various medical conditions.

Chapter 3 - The Benefits of Hydrogen Therapy

In recent times, hydrogen therapy has garnered interest due to its promising health benefits, particularly for adults and the elderly. Due to its tiny molecular size, H2 can seamlessly traverse cell membranes and even cross the blood-brain barrier, effectively neutralizing harmful free radicals in the brain.

Understanding the Benefits of Hydrogen Gas Therapy

- Improves Weight Loss
- Reduces Oxidative Stress in the Body
- Improves Insulin Sensitivity
- Improves Fasting Blood Glucose
- Reduces Blood Pressure
- Improves Diabetic Neuropathy
- Offers Neuroprotective Benefits
- Improves Visual Function.
- Reduces Insulin Resistance
- Reduces Brain Damage due to Stroke.

https://www.ncbi.nlm.nih.gov/pmc/articles/PMC8956398/

How Hydrogen Supports Cellular Health

At the most basic level, our bodies are made up of trillions of cells, each carrying out essential functions to keep us alive and healthy. Free radicals can expedite aging and up the risk of chronic diseases. Hydrogen's knack for neutralizing these radicals makes it a prospective instrument for cellular rejuvenation. By neutralizing these free radicals, hydrogen acts as a powerful antioxidant, protecting our cells from oxidative stress and promoting cellular health.

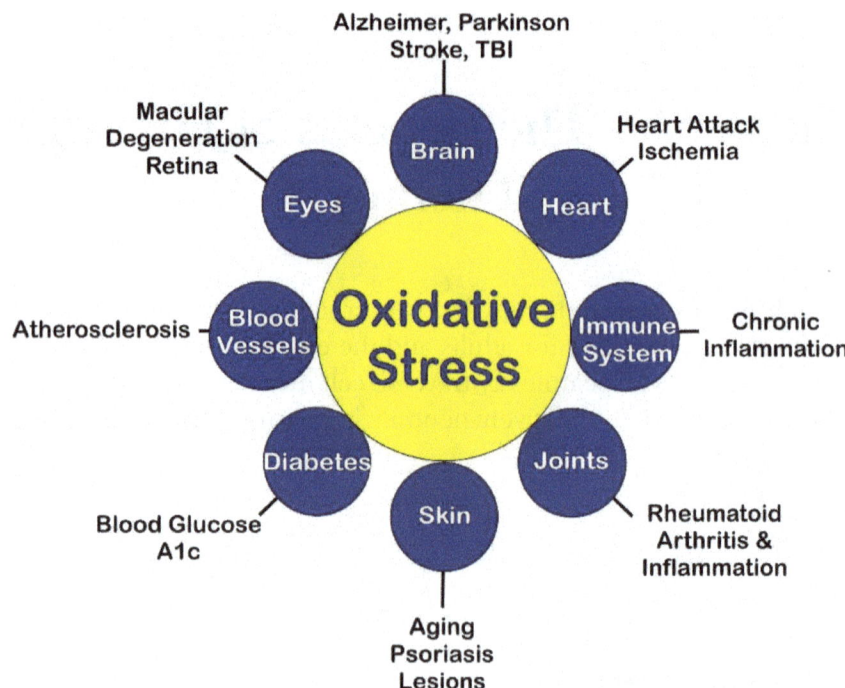

Young or old, inflammation is a natural response of the immune system to injury or infection. However, chronic inflammation can contribute to the development of numerous diseases, including cardiovascular problems, arthritis, and even cancer. Studies have shown that hydrogen can suppress the production of pro-inflammatory molecules, thus reducing inflammation and potentially alleviating the symptoms associated with these conditions.

Molecular hydrogen uniquely acts as a selective antioxidant, targeting specifically the harmful hydroxyl radicals ($\cdot$OH), while preserving beneficial radicals such as nitric oxide (NO). Additionally, hydrogen has been shown to activate the NRF2 pathway, a critical biological mechanism that stimulates the body's natural production of internal antioxidants, including glutathione and superoxide dismutase. These antioxidants significantly reduce oxidative stress and inflammation, thereby promoting cellular health and protecting tissues from oxidative damage. Further information on the NRF2 pathway and its role can be explored here:

Hydrogen's Antioxidant Properties

Antioxidants play a crucial role in safeguarding our bodies against the damaging effects of free radicals. Free radicals are unstable molecules that can cause oxidative stress, leading to cell damage and various health issues and are linked to aging. Hydrogen Gas Therapy acts as a potent antioxidant by neutralizing free radicals, helping to protect our cells and tissues from harm.

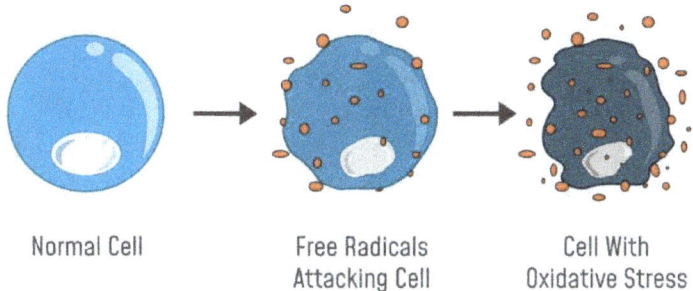

Role of H2 Infused Water in Energy Production

Enhance mitochondrial function.

Mitochondria are the powerhouses of our cells, responsible for producing the energy needed for cellular activities. As we age, mitochondrial function naturally declines, leading to decreased energy production and increased fatigue. Hydrogen therapy has been shown to improve mitochondrial function, potentially boosting energy levels and overall vitality in adults and seniors.

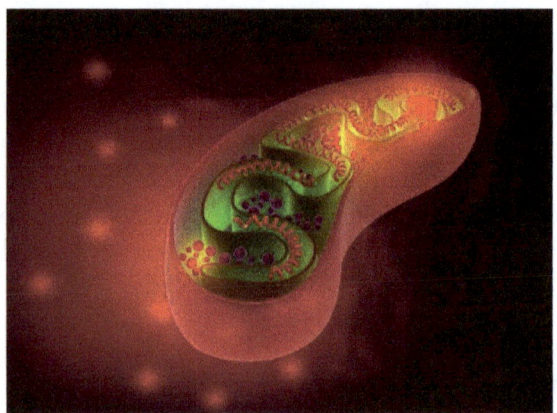

Hydrogen Gas has been found beneficial in the mitochondria's production of adenosine triphosphate (ATP), the energy currency of our cells. ATP provides energy for various cellular processes, including muscle contraction, nerve signaling, and metabolism. Hydrogen ions are involved in the electron transport chain for critical enzymes that convert glucose into ATP, ensuring a steady energy supply.

Adenosine triphospate (ATP)

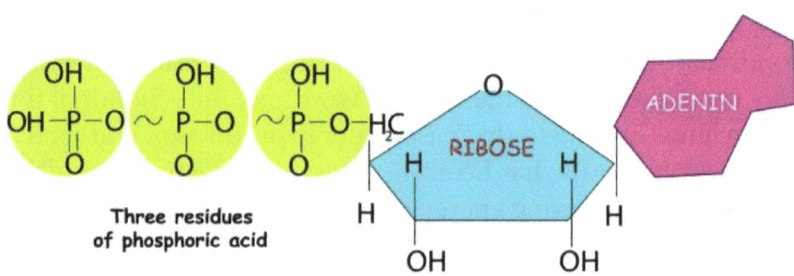

Chapter 4 - Maximize Your Experience

Using This Book

This guide dives into hydrogen therapy, elucidating how it can bolster health, sharpen cognitive function, lift energy levels, and foster overall well-being. For those keen on anti-aging, hydrogen's capacity to neutralize free radicals and curtail cellular damage suggests it may slow the aging process.

Clinical Observations on Hydrogen Therapy

Medical studies available in PubMed indicate that hydrogen gas therapy not only reduces inflammation but also improves cognitive function and enhances athletic performance. Hydrogen-infused water also boasts antioxidant properties, promoting cellular health and offering protection against age-related decline.

Maximizing Your Experience

1. **Approach with a Skeptical Mind:** Cross-referencing content with resources is paramount. Everyone's response to therapy varies, and while hydrogen therapy might be novel to some, its foundational science isn't.
2. **Seek Professional Guidance:** Consult healthcare professionals before adopting hydrogen therapy, ensuring personalized and optimal results.
3. **Experiment and Implement:** After absorbing this book, you might consider trying some recommendations.
4. **Connect with Others:** Engage in communities or online forums, like certain Facebook groups, centered around hydrogen therapy to gain diverse insights.

A Modest Effect

It's easy to hype the effect of hydrogen therapy and infused water, and it is not intentional. It happens by reporting on the positive effects of scientific studies on the biological effects of hydrogen. The positive effects reported are not anecdotal. People are not drinking hydrogen-infused water and telling researchers it makes them feel better. The biological effects require scientific instruments to measure and confirm the positive results.

Modest is an important concept. People jump from one fad to the next, when immediate expectations in their physiology do not occur. The effects are modest, and unless you are measuring the results scientifically in double-blind experiments, you could easily miss its effect.

Modest doesn't mean the effect isn't there, it just isn't obvious.

The positive effects may be subtle, like supplementing with vitamins. Unless you are addressing a vitamin deficiency, supplements will rarely result in a noticeable, immediate positive change. However, over the long run, vitamins will result in being healthier.

When I drink hydrogen-infused water, I do not notice any immediate effect. However, the one immediate benefit is that I am drinking 16-24 oz of water per day that I usually would not drink, and even at that baseline level, it improves my hydration. The additional benefits of the H2 gas infused in the water are chronicled in the studies shown in this book. Just know the effects are subtle, and benefits are obtained over time.

Your body, through the digestive process, generates hydrogen gas. Well, the microbiome in your digestive tract generates hydrogen gas. We expel this gas as farts. Ingesting hydrogen gas does provide the body with additional hydrogen gas. Now that I have cleared the air of expectations, we can move forward.

Remember: while hydrogen therapies offer promising complementary health benefits, they shouldn't supplant conventional medical treatments. Nonetheless, their potential to elevate overall well-being makes them worthy additions to any health regimen.

Complementing H2 with Red Light Therapy

Many of the positive observations made with H2 gas, specifically improved mitochondrial function, have also been observed with Red Light Therapy, also called photobiomodulation (PBM). I've written on RLT available on Amazon.
https://www.amazon.com/Living-Younger-Longer-Light-Therapy-ebook/dp/B09FC59M4Z

Interestingly, RLT is also used to treat neurodegenerative diseases and dysfunction. One 2021 study applied both treatments of RLT and H2 to achieve remarkable results with Parkinson patients.

https://www.ncbi.nlm.nih.gov/pmc/articles/PMC7850666

Improvements from the baseline were noted in a week. The study concluded that PBM + H2 reduced the severity of the disease and called for more and larger clinical studies.

Synergy (H2 + RLT + ALA)

Hydrogen Gas is one of three current treatments that produce positive, modest, but measurable scientific results. I have noted the improvement in Parkinson's disease by combining Red Light Therapy (RLT) with H2, but there is a third supplement, Alpha Lipoic Acid (ALA).

I have written a pamphlet on the benefits of Alpha Lipoic Acid, that is available on Amazon.com.

https://www.amazon.com/dp/B0CH5PHXW1

All these therapies boost the aging mitochondria's function. ALA supplements, like Hydrogen, are a powerful antioxidant. If a person took ALA supplements, combined with hydrogen therapy and RLT, would the combination create a potent synergic treatment option?

This is a question I hope will be answered soon with clinical studies.

Chapter 5 - Is Hydrogen Gas Therapy Safe?

Hydrogen gas is colorless, odorless, and tasteless. When hydrogen is infused in water under pressure, it becomes like carbonated water, with the exception that the gas dissolved in the water is hydrogen, not carbon dioxide as in standard soda pop.

The concentration of hydrogen gas dissolved in water is typically between 0.5 mg/L (ppm) to 1.5 mg/L (ppm). The concentration of dissolved hydrogen in water will be covered more deeply in the water ionizer section.

As stated, hydrogen gas is created naturally in our gut by anaerobic digestion. In one study, a maximum of 1.5 liters of gas can be produced by gut bacteria in a day.

https://www.sciencedirect.com/science/article/pii/S1756464622004376

Hydrogen gas is non-toxic. Hydrogen therapy is considered safe for all age groups.

Hydrogen gas is flammable. This isn't a concern for people using H2-infused water. However, it is a consideration for people with machines generating high flow rates (120 to 240 mL/min) of H2 gas for inhaling. If the H2 gas is allowed to accumulate to an appreciable volume, it may become dangerous. Hydrogen gas, mixed with air, can be ignited from a spark or flame.

Potential Interactions with Medications: Always consult with a healthcare professional regarding potential interactions between hydrogen-infused water and medications. Some drugs might be affected by the water in terms of absorption or metabolism. Seniors especially need to be cautious due to potential variations in drug processing.

FDA Ruling on Hydrogen Safety

The FDA has ruled that hydrogen water containing no more than 2.14% solubilized molecular hydrogen is Generally Recognized as Safe (GRAS). This ruling allows up to two liters of H2-infused water to be consumed daily (FDA, Agency Response Letter GRAS Notice No. 520

While molecular hydrogen is considered safe and well-tolerated, it is essential to consult with your healthcare provider before introducing it alongside your current medications. Currently, there is limited scientific evidence specifically addressing the effects of molecular hydrogen on pregnant and nursing women.

H2 gas provides a therapeutic effect and is not toxic to the liver or kidneys.

Overconsumption of Water

I am more concerned about the overconsumption of water, which can cause a condition called water toxicity. The United States CDC recommends NOT drinking more than 48 ounces of water per day. Recently, actress Brook Shields had grand mal seizures from the overconsumption of water in preparation for her one-woman show.

https://nypost.com/2023/11/02/lifestyle/drinking-too-much-water-can-cause-seizures-brooke-shields-health-scare-explained/

Chapter 6 - Hydrogen Wellness for Seniors

As we age, our bodies accumulate free radicals, which can lead to oxidative stress and damage cells. Hydrogen acts as a selective antioxidant, neutralizing these harmful free radicals and reducing oxidative stress. This can result in improved cellular health, reduced inflammation, and enhanced immune function.

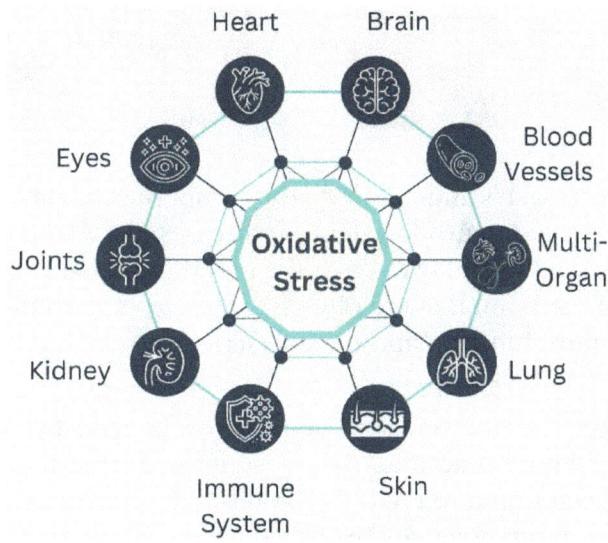

Hydrogen therapy may help seniors more. This study shows that H2-infused water made significant improvements in the BAP (biological antioxidant potential) of people older than 30 but not in the younger participants.

https://www.ncbi.nlm.nih.gov/pmc/articles/PMC7376192/

Improved Cognitive Function

Oxidative stress and chronic inflammation are known to contribute to cognitive decline and neurodegenerative diseases, such as Alzheimer's and Parkinson's.

Hydrogen gas and hydrogen-infused water have been linked to notable improvements in cognitive function. The potential benefits stem from hydrogen's ability to neutralize harmful free radicals in the brain. This neutralization helps mitigate oxidative stress, which can contribute to cognitive decline. As a result, hydrogen supports the neurons, leading to enhanced cognitive performance.

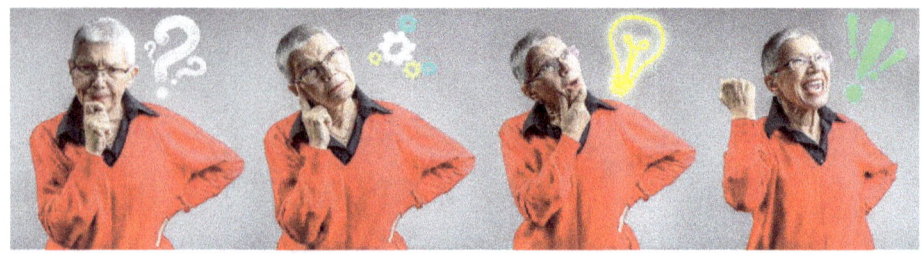

Additionally, hydrogen's anti-inflammatory properties might be valuable in combating age-related neurodegenerative diseases like Alzheimer's and Parkinson's. Its unique ability to cross the blood-brain barrier allows it to benefit areas of the brain that are often hard to target, thereby directly enhancing cognitive function and mental clarity.

Seniors and athletes can leverage these cognitive benefits by integrating hydrogen-infused water into their daily regimens. Furthermore, molecular hydrogen has been found to cross the blood-brain barrier easily, allowing it to directly access brain tissue and exert its beneficial effects. Once inside the brain, it can help regulate neurotransmitter levels, promoting better communication between brain cells and enhancing cognitive function.

Studies have demonstrated that molecular hydrogen supplementation can improve memory, attention, and overall mental clarity.

Clinical Evidence Supporting Hydrogen Therapy in Seniors

Clinical evidence further supports hydrogen therapy's efficacy, particularly among elderly populations. A notable study conducted during the COVID-19 lockdowns observed elderly adults aged 70 and above consuming hydrogen-infused water. Results showed a remarkable 4% increase in telomere length—a significant marker associated with reduced aging and improved cellular health. Participants also reported improvements in sleep quality and enhanced mobility, objectively measured using a "sit-to-stand" performance test. Moreover, despite experiencing significant stress and immobility, participants showed reduced inflammation markers, specifically C-reactive protein (CRP), and improved cardiovascular function. Details of this clinical study can be further reviewed at :

https://www.sciencedirect.com/science/article/abs/pii/S0531556521003569

Hydrogen Gas Improves Brain Function in Alzheimer's Patients

Significant improvements in Alzheimer's patients have been confirmed with clinical studies.

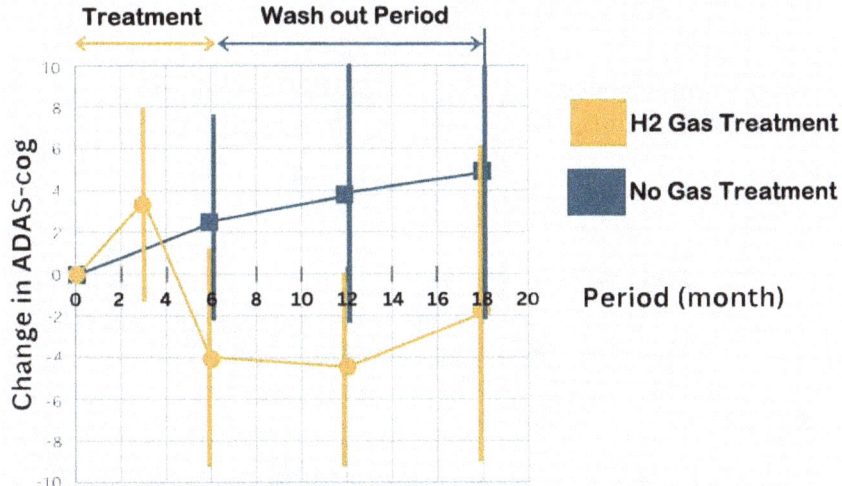

Alzheimer's Disease Assessment Scale-cognitive subscale (ADAS-cog)
Chart based on information in the following clinical study.

https://www.ncbi.nlm.nih.gov/pmc/articles/PMC10057981/

The H2-treated group inhaled 3% H2 gas for 1 hour twice a day for 6 months. The staff administering the ADAS-cog test were unaware of which participants were in the treated or untreated group. A lower value in the ADAS-cog indicates an improvement, while a higher score indicates a worse outcome. Researchers believe the initial worsening of the treated H2 gas group may have been due to the stress of wearing a face mask. After three months, the treated group showed significant improvement and maintained this improvement for a considerable amount of time during the washout period with H2 gas supplementation.

The untreated group continually worsened, as was expected.

https://pubmed.ncbi.nlm.nih.gov/36986533/

Molecular Hydrogen in Drinking Water Protects against Neurodegenerative Changes Induced by Traumatic Brain Injury

https://journals.plos.org/plosone/article?id=10.1371/journal.pone.0108034

Quantification of hydrogen production by intestinal bacteria that are specifically dysregulated in Parkinson's disease.

https://journals.plos.org/plosone/article?id=10.1371/journal.pone.0208313

Interestingly, some studies show that H2-infused water improves the individual gut microbiome, which improves neurodegenerative diseases.

Boosting Energy Levels and Vitality

Hydrogen is not just a cognitive booster but also a potent energy enhancer. It supports the body's natural metabolic processes and cellular energy production. Whether through drinking hydrogen-infused water or inhaling hydrogen gas, the resulting energy boost can help seniors reclaim vitality, aid athletes in elevating their performance, and assist individuals in unlocking their potential.

Drinking hydrogen water enhances endurance and relieves psychometric fatigue: a randomized, double-blind, placebo-controlled study
https://pubmed.ncbi.nlm.nih.gov/31251888/

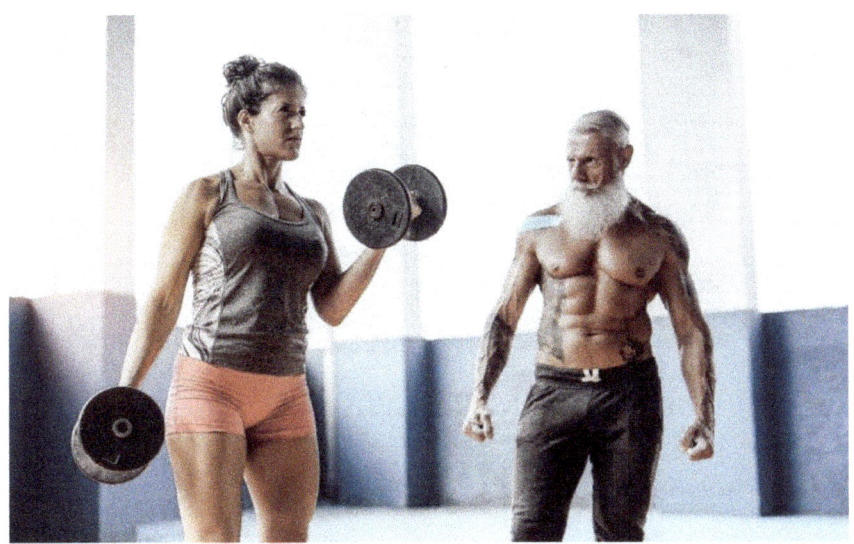

The following study shows how H2 boosts recovery after exercise.

https://pubmed.ncbi.nlm.nih.gov/30243702/

Supporting Cardiovascular Health

Another significant benefit of hydrogen therapy is its potential to improve cardiovascular health. Hydrogen has been shown to have anti-inflammatory and anti-apoptotic effects on the heart, reducing the risk of cardiovascular diseases such as hypertension, atherosclerosis, and heart failure.

Hydrogen gas holds promise in managing cholesterol levels. Elevated LDL cholesterol can result in plaque buildup in arteries, increasing the risk of heart attacks or strokes. Hydrogen gas might help lower these LDL cholesterol levels, promoting artery health and decreasing cardiovascular risks. Particularly for seniors, the flexibility of blood vessels can decrease with age, making the cardiovascular benefits of hydrogen especially pertinent.

Age-Related Macular Degeneration

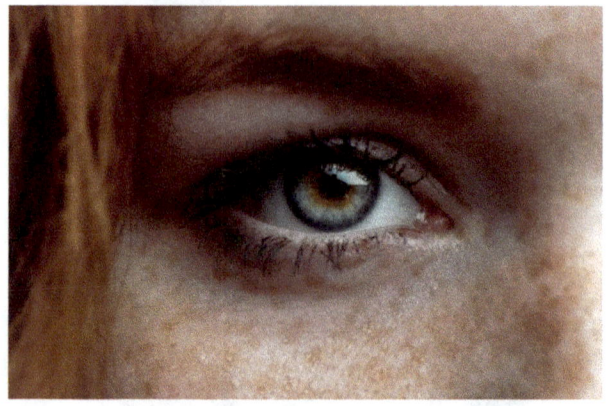

https://www.ncbi.nlm.nih.gov/pmc/articles/PMC8584469/

Strengthening the Immune System

Hydrogen's antioxidant properties make it a robust tool for bolstering the immune system. Its capacity to counteract harmful free radicals diminishes oxidative stress and inflammation, factors that can weaken the immune response. Hydrogen gas therapy has been spotlighted for its potential to modulate the immune system, improving its resilience against infections and diseases. Some studies even suggest it might help decelerate the aging process.

Promoting Joint Health and Reducing Inflammation

Hydrogen's antioxidant capabilities extend to joint health. By neutralizing free radicals, it may prevent joint tissue degradation and alleviate symptoms related to conditions such as osteoarthritis.

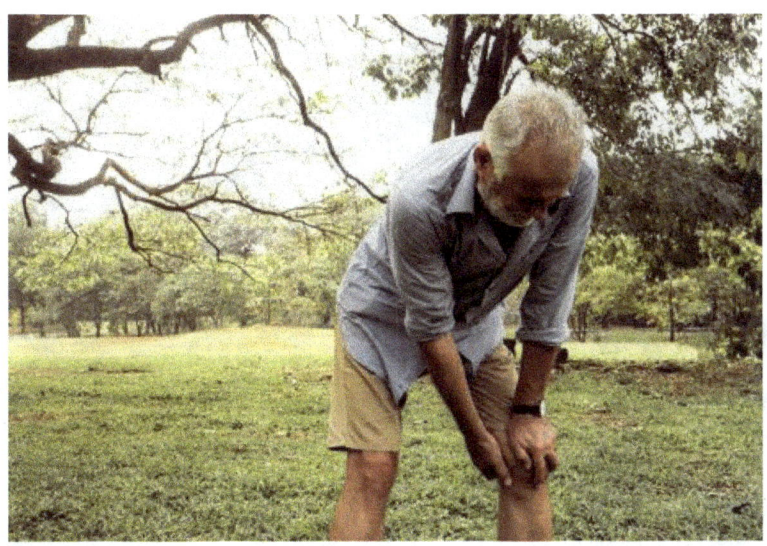

Senior Exercise

Hydrogen has been shown to enhance exercise performance by reducing fatigue and improving muscle function. This can be advantageous for seniors who may experience muscle weakness or fatigue during physical activities.

Hydrogen therapy can increase endurance, improve recovery time, and allow for more enjoyable and effective workouts.

By reducing oxidative stress and inflammation, hydrogen therapy can aid in faster recovery, reduce muscle soreness, and improve overall athletic performance. For seniors looking to maintain an active lifestyle, hydrogen therapy can be particularly beneficial.

https://www.ncbi.nlm.nih.gov/pmc/articles/PMC8092150/

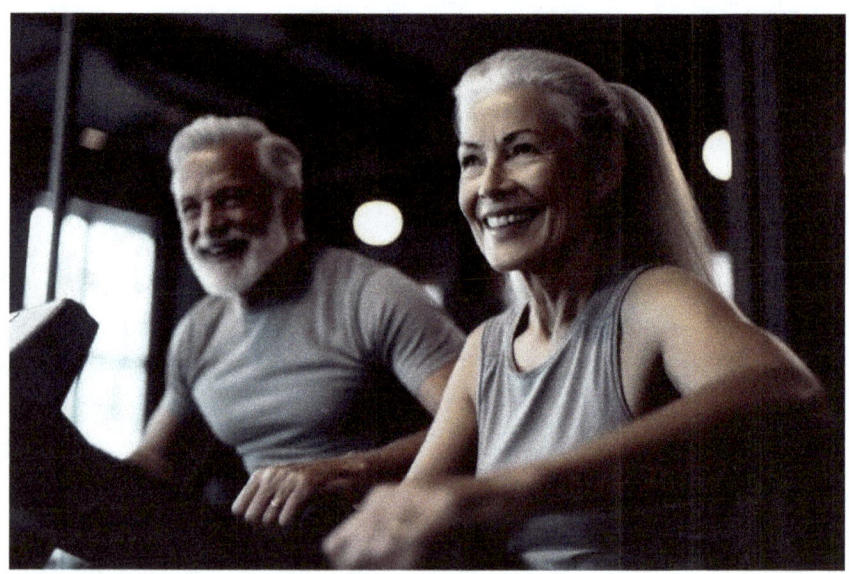

Metabolic Syndrome

Studies show that H2-infused water reduces oxidative stress related to Metabolic Syndrome.

https://www.ncbi.nlm.nih.gov/pmc/articles/PMC3679390/

This 24-week study showed significant reductions in blood cholesterol, blood glucose, A1c, and improved biomarkers for inflammation in the H2-infused water group. The researchers also noted a slight reduction in body mass index. The daily amount of H2 ingested was 5.5 millimoles daily. If I have my math correct, that is about 11mg/h2. To achieve this dosage, the researchers used H2 tablets, 3X daily in 250 ml of water.

https://www.ncbi.nlm.nih.gov/pmc/articles/PMC7102907/

Aiding in Digestion and Gut Health

Hydrogen gas contributes to a balanced gut microbiome, essential for digestion, nutrient absorption, immune function, and mood regulation. An imbalanced microbiome can manifest as bloating, constipation, or other digestive issues.

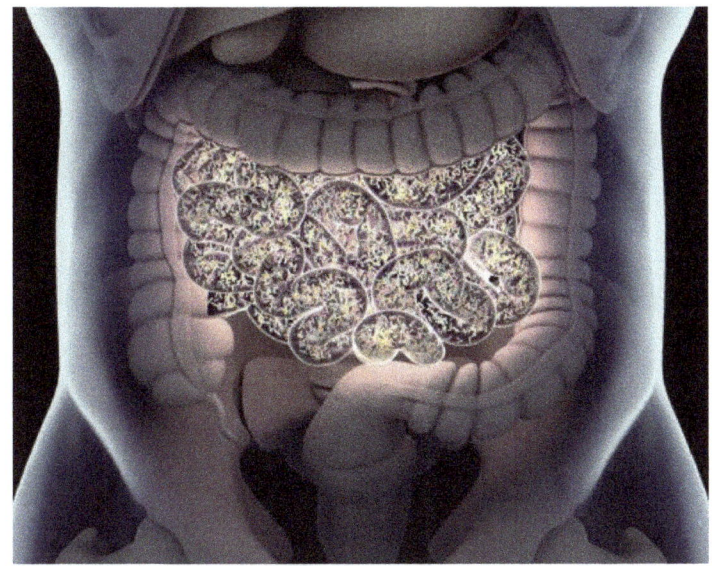

Especially for seniors, whose digestive systems might be more prone to inflammation and oxidative stress, hydrogen-infused water can be a remedy. Athletes, too, after intense workouts, can benefit from hydrogen's positive effects on digestion.

Improving Sleep Quality and Managing Stress

In our fast-paced world, quality sleep and stress management are paramount. Hydrogen-infused water and hydrogen gas, with their antioxidant and anti-inflammatory properties, can counteract the physiological impacts of stress. By adding hydrogen to their routine, individuals might experience relaxation, reduced anxiety, and better sleep.

Establishing a regular sleep schedule and relaxing pre-sleep rituals can enhance sleep quality. Chronic stress can be detrimental to health, but hydrogen's properties defend against its negative effects.

In conclusion, hydrogen's myriad benefits present a compelling case for its inclusion in daily wellness routines. Whether you're a senior, an athlete, or simply someone seeking improved health, the advantages of hydrogen can be transformative.

Chapter 7 - Hydrogen for Athletes

Athletic Advantages

Athletes might find hydrogen particularly beneficial. Research suggests hydrogen can ameliorate exercise-induced fatigue, facilitate recovery, and uplift performance[2]. The reduction of oxidative stress and inflammation means enhanced endurance and prowess.

https://pubmed.ncbi.nlm.nih.gov/31574544/

Athletes and fitness enthusiasts drink hydrogen-infused water before a workout, which can help protect your cells from damage and promote faster recovery.

One of the primary benefits of hydrogen therapy for athletes is its ability to enhance endurance. Studies have shown that hydrogen-rich water can delay the onset of fatigue and improve stamina. By increasing the body's antioxidant capacity, hydrogen therapy allows athletes to push their limits, leading to longer training sessions and improved performance.

Additionally, hydrogen therapy has been found to accelerate post-exercise recovery.

Intense workouts often result in muscle soreness and damage. However, hydrogen-rich water has been shown to alleviate these symptoms by reducing inflammation and promoting tissue repair. This enables athletes to bounce back quicker and train more frequently, leading to greater gains in strength and overall performance.

Mental clarity and focus are crucial for athletes, and hydrogen-rich water has demonstrated the potential to enhance cognitive performance. By reducing oxidative stress in the brain, hydrogen therapy may improve reaction times, decision-making abilities, and overall mental acuity, allowing athletes to stay sharp during intense competition.

It is important to note that hydrogen therapy should be complemented with a well-rounded training program and a balanced diet. While hydrogen therapy can undoubtedly enhance athletic performance, it is not a substitute for proper training and nutrition. Athletes should also consult with their healthcare provider before incorporating hydrogen therapy into their routine, as individual needs may vary.

Intense Exercise & Recovery

During intense physical activity, the body produces reactive oxygen species (ROS). These ROS can lead to oxidative stress, inflammation, and muscle fatigue. Hydrogen molecules can selectively neutralize these harmful ROS. By adopting hydrogen-infused water or hydrogen gas inhalation, athletes might experience enhanced endurance, quicker energy replenishment, and improved post-workout recovery. Hydrogen also reduces lactic acid accumulation, which is associated with muscle soreness.

Engaging in vigorous activities like sprinting or high jumps can cause an uptick in free radicals, which may result in oxidative stress, potentially causing muscle harm and swelling.

One involving ten male soccer players averaging 21 years in age, it was found that consuming 500 mL (approximately 17 fluid ounces) of hydrogen water the evening prior, along with two additional 500 mL portions on the day of physical testing, helped lower post-exercise blood lactate concentrations and reduced certain muscle fatigue indicators when compared to placebo water. The hydrogen concentration in the water was about 1 mM (roughly 2 ppm).

https://pubmed.ncbi.nlm.nih.gov/22520831/

Testosterone Production.

Researchers are beginning to investigate improved testosterone production for infertility, sperm motility, radiation damage, testicular injury, erectile dysfunction, spinal cord hemi section-induced testicular injury, testicular torsion, etc.

For women: osteoporosis after menopause, premature ovarian failure, uterine inflammation, breast cancer, etc.

https://www.ncbi.nlm.nih.gov/pmc/articles/PMC7826209/

Hydrogen acts like an Antioxidant and Anti-inflammatory for Rheumatoid Arthritis

https://www.ncbi.nlm.nih.gov/pmc/articles/PMC3788323/

Drinking 500 ml of H2 infused water daily for 4 weeks significantly improved patients Rheumatoid Arthritis

Chapter 8 - Anti-Aging

Anti-Aging Attributes

As we age, cellular function naturally declines, leading to a variety of health issues. The anti-aging sector is optimistic about hydrogen's potential to improve cellular function and energy production. Studies show hydrogen shields cellular DNA, boosts mitochondrial function, and regulates gene expression—all of which result in increased vitality and stamina, and decelerate aging, and foster longevity.

When hydrogen is introduced into the body, it acts as a powerful antioxidant, neutralizing harmful free radicals that contribute to aging and various age-related diseases.

Role of Molecular Hydrogen in Ageing and Ageing-Related Diseases" by Zhiling Fu, Jin Zhang, and Yan Zhang
https://www.ncbi.nlm.nih.gov/pmc/articles/PMC8956398/

Research has shown that hydrogen therapy can enhance cellular function and reduce oxidative stress, a key factor in aging. By reducing oxidative stress, hydrogen therapy helps protect our DNA, proteins, and lipids from damage, which ultimately leads to a more youthful appearance and improved overall health.

Furthermore, hydrogen therapy has been found to have a positive impact on various age-related conditions. For instance, it can help improve cognitive function and memory, which often decline with age. Hydrogen therapy also promotes cardiovascular health by reducing inflammation and oxidative stress, thus lowering the risk of heart disease and stroke.

Anti-Aging and Hydrogen

Aging is often accompanied by oxidative stress, inflammation, and cognitive decline. Hydrogen therapy might counteract these effects. Research suggests it can improve cognitive performance, memory, and overall brain health.

Additionally, by reducing inflammation, hydrogen therapy can aid muscle recovery, which is beneficial for seniors and athletes alike. It's a promising tool in the anti-aging toolkit, but more research is needed. Always consult with healthcare experts before starting any hydrogen therapy.

Animal Studies - I like animal studies because animals are less vulnerable to the placebo effect.

https://www.ncbi.nlm.nih.gov/pmc/articles/PMC6235982/

Animal studies have shown that supplementation with molecular hydrogen can increase the lifespan of organisms such as fruit flies and worms by up to 30%. While more research is needed, these findings hold promise for humans as well. While more research is needed, these findings hold promise for humans as well.

Chapter 9 - Hydrogen For Chronic Illness

Recent progress toward hydrogen medicine: the potential of molecular hydrogen for preventive and therapeutic applications.
https://pubmed.ncbi.nlm.nih.gov/21736547/

Hydrogen's Potential in Diabetes Management

Emerging research suggests that hydrogen might have a role to play in diabetes management.

Molecular hydrogen improves type 2 diabetes through inhibiting oxidative stress.
https://pubmed.ncbi.nlm.nih.gov/32537002/

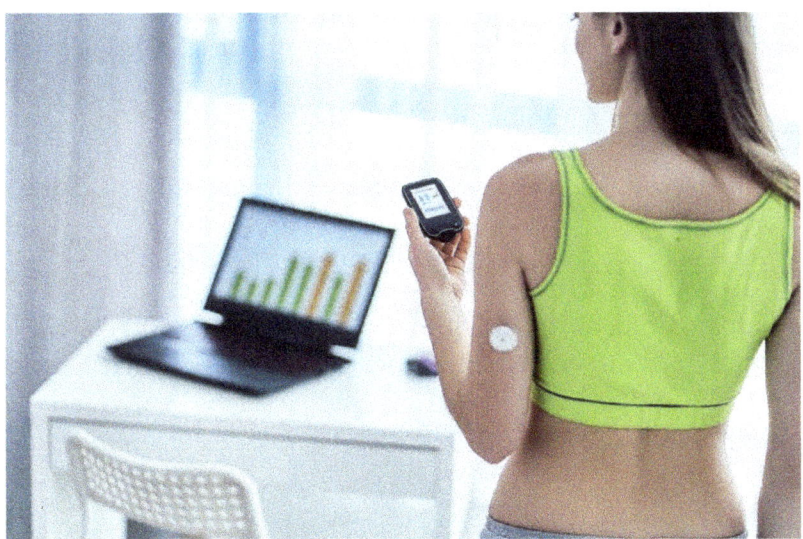

One study explored the impact of consuming H2-infused water on people with type 2 diabetes mellitus (T2DM) and those with impaired glucose tolerance (IGT). The investigator required the 36 participants to drink 900ml of either hydrogen-infused or placebo water daily for an initial eight-week period. Followed by a 12-week wash-out phase. The participant then completes a second eight-week period of drinking the other type of water. Outcomes indicated that the hydrogen-enriched water markedly decreased oxidative stress, lowered LDL cholesterol, and enhanced insulin sensitivity. Additionally, it elevated levels of adiponectin and EC-SOD, both beneficial for glucose and lipid regulation. Impressively, after undergoing the hydrogen water regimen, four of the six individuals with IGT returned to normal glucose tolerance levels. These insights point to the potential of hydrogen-rich water as a therapeutic aid in diabetes management and possibly in deterring the development of T2DM.

https://bioresonancetherapy.com/articles/hydrogen-water-reduce-risk-of-type-2-diabetes-with-simple-change/

H2 Drops Blood Glucose -20 points, A1C down 12%

Researchers enrolled 60 participants in a 24-week study and observed significant reductions in Fasting Blood Glucose (FBG) and A1C.
https://www.ncbi.nlm.nih.gov/pmc/articles/PMC7102907/

Supplementation of hydrogen-rich water improves lipid and glucose metabolism in patients with type 2 diabetes or impaired glucose tolerance

https://pubmed.ncbi.nlm.nih.gov/19083400/

Molecular hydrogen improves type 2 diabetes by inhibiting oxidative stress.

https://www.ncbi.nlm.nih.gov/pmc/articles/PMC7291681/

Supplementation of hydrogen-rich water improves lipid and glucose metabolism in patients with type 2 diabetes or impaired glucose tolerance.

https://www.sciencedirect.com/science/article/abs/pii/S0271531708000237

Clinical Studies on Prediabetes and Metabolic

Syndrome

Specific Clinical Results (Prediabetes Trial)

In one controlled study, participants with early-stage glucose intolerance consumed approximately 900 mL of hydrogen-infused water each day for eight weeks. Nearly two-thirds achieved normal glucose tolerance levels, accompanied by reductions in oxidative stress markers. Four out of six individuals with impaired glucose tolerance normalized their oral glucose tolerance test results. The intervention also lowered modified LDL cholesterol, small dense LDL, and urinary 8-isoprostanes, and increased levels of extracellular superoxide dismutase and adiponectin.

https://pubmed.ncbi.nlm.nih.gov/19083400/

Metabolic Syndrome Study Specifics

Another pilot study involving 20 individuals with metabolic syndrome markers reported:

- A ~39% increase in antioxidant enzyme (superoxide dismutase, SOD) activity.
- A ~43% reduction in lipid peroxidation (measured by TBARS).
- An ~8% rise in HDL cholesterol and a 13% reduction in total/HDL cholesterol ratio, with no change in fasting glucose levels.

https://pmc.ncbi.nlm.nih.gov/articles/PMC2831093

Animal Studies Insights

In type 1 diabetic mouse models, chronic hydrogen water intake significantly reduced blood sugar levels and preserved insulin-producing beta cells. Other rodent studies demonstrate improved muscle glucose uptake, attributed to an increase in GLUT4 transporter movement to cell surfaces—even with low insulin presence.
https://john-iovine.medium.com/can-hydrogen-water-help-tame-your-blood-sugar-87acf8addcdf

Mechanisms Explained Simply

Molecular hydrogen appears to neutralize harmful free radicals, protecting pancreatic and vascular tissues. It also modulates inflammatory signaling pathways—including NF-κB—and supports insulin-independent muscle glucose uptake by amplifying GLUT4 transporter activity.
https://en.wikipedia.org/wiki/Hydrogen_therapy

Practical Recommendations for Consumers

Hydrogen infusers—such as electrolysis-based devices commonly sold online—are practical for home use. For an 8-ounce serving, a five-minute infusion with immediate consumption is recommended to retain hydrogen before it dissipates. Users should monitor markers like oxidative stress and cholesterol before expecting changes in fasting glucose and allow about 8–12 weeks for evaluation.

Clear Advisory for Consumers

It is vital to emphasize that hydrogen water should be used as a supplement—not a replacement—for established diabetes treatments (diet, medications, insulin, and exercise). Hydrogen water is best considered as a supportive, complementary approach alongside conventional medical care.

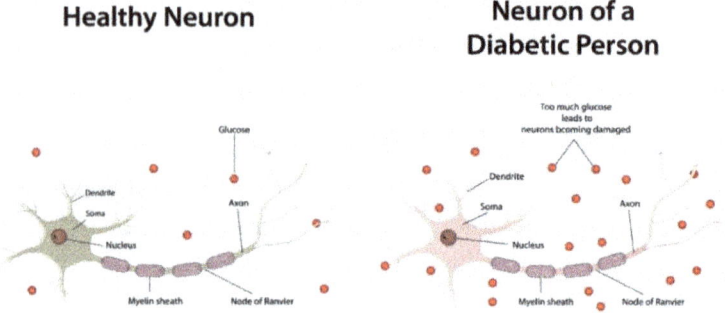

Improves Diabetic Neuropath.

Weight Loss

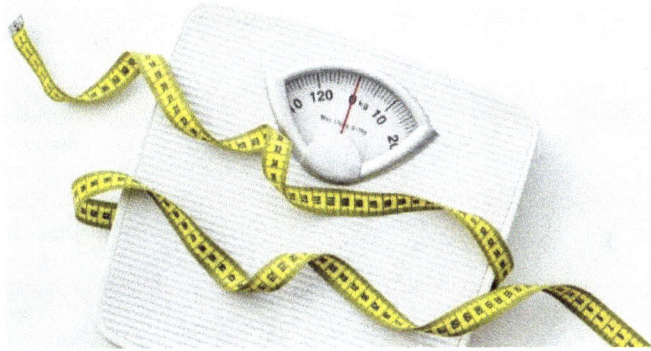

The following study is an animal study with mice, that improves not only obesity but diabetes as well.

https://pubmed.ncbi.nlm.nih.gov/21293445/

There is also anecdotal information from researchers and people who claim H2 therapy and H2-infused water helps significantly with fat loss.

https://www.yahoo.com/lifestyle/hydrogen-infused-water-key-weight-150724362.html

Improves Retinal Degeneration

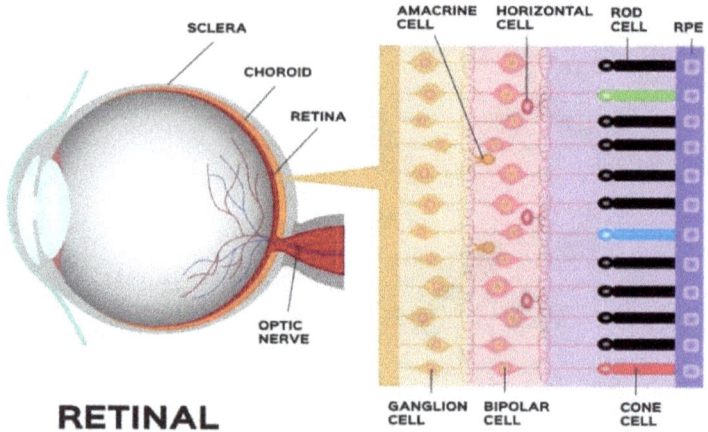

https://www.ophthalmologytimes.com/view/arvo-2023-hydrogen-rich-water-in-the-treatment-of-retinal-degeneration

Hydrogen-infused water helps rejuvenate skin.

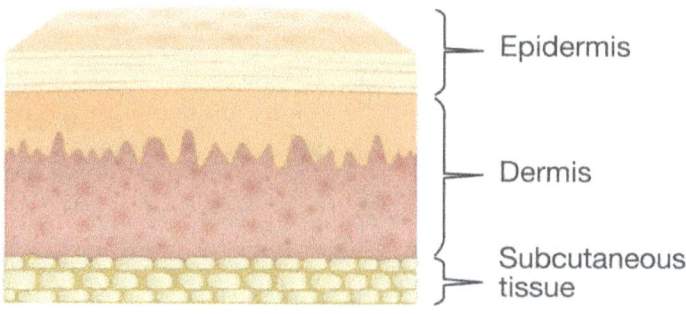

https://pubmed.ncbi.nlm.nih.gov/22070900/

Hydrogen Anti-Inflammatory for Rheumatoid Arthritis

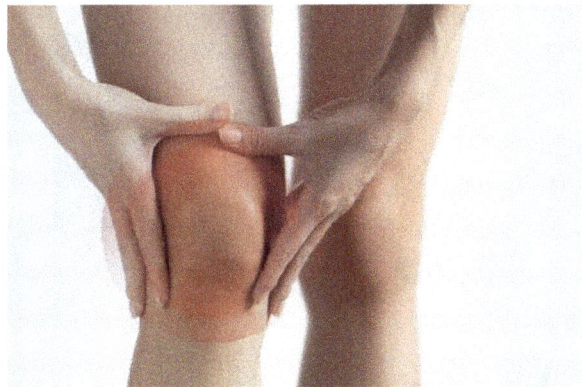

https://www.ncbi.nlm.nih.gov/pmc/articles/PMC3788323/

Drinking 500 ml of high H2-infused water daily for four weeks significantly improved patient's Rheumatoid Arthritis.

Better than Caffeine

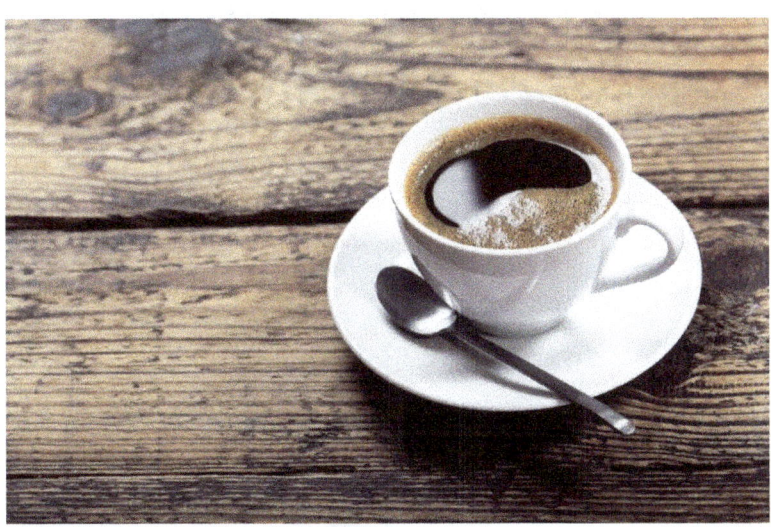

Hydrogen-rich water (HRW) is more effective than caffeine at improving brain metabolism and alertness in sleep-deprived individuals.

https://onlinelibrary.wiley.com/doi/10.1002/fsn3.2480#fsn32480-bib-0024

Blood Pressure

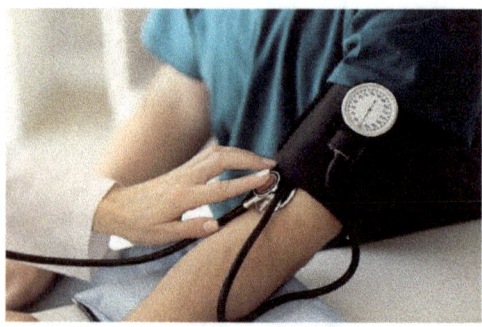

Improvements in blood pressure are preliminary. This is a rat study using H2 gas inhalation. The positive result beacons a need for human clinical trials.

https://www.nature.com/articles/s41598-020-77349-8lin

H2-Infused Water Reduces Impact of Chemotherapy

Cancer patients given H2-infused water have significantly less damage to their liver from chemotherapy than a control group given plain water.

https://pubmed.ncbi.nlm.nih.gov/29142752/

Chapter 10 – Hydrogen For Eye Health

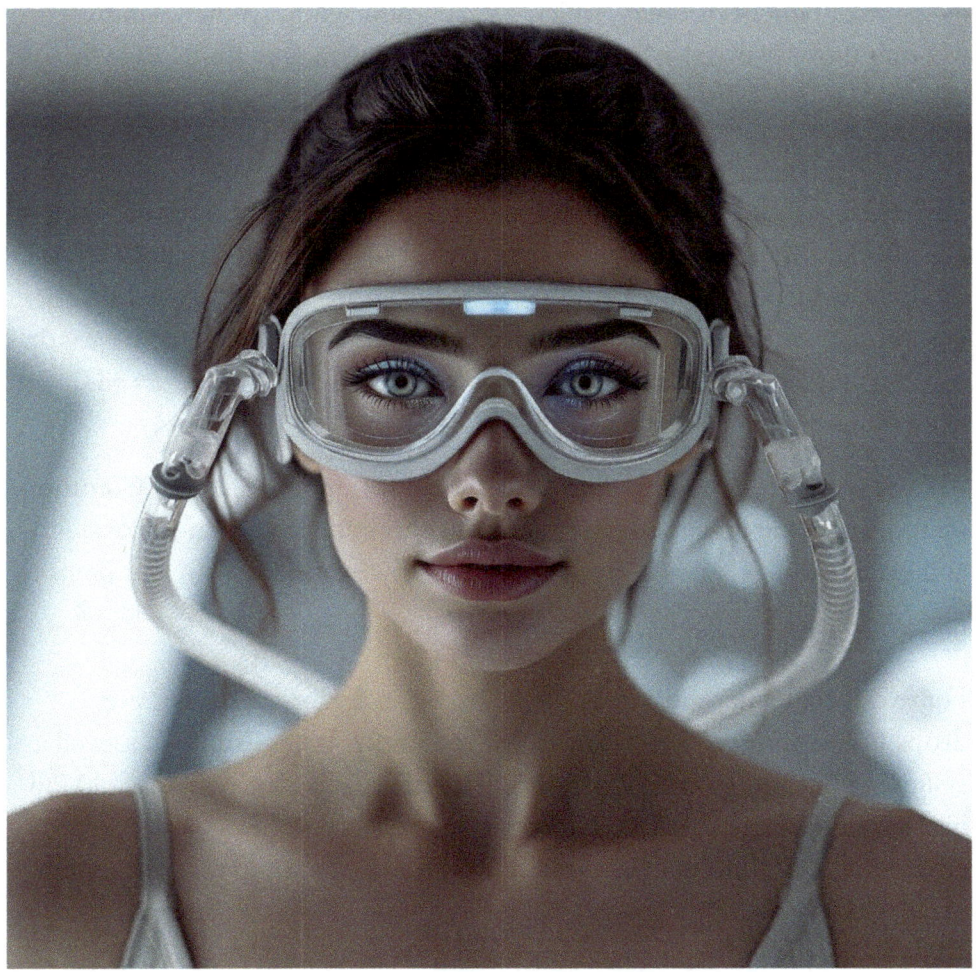

For eye health, some companies are beginning to market **hydrogen-delivery goggles** — devices that channel Hydrogen gas (often generated from water via electrolysis) to bathe the eyes in H2 gas.

The idea is that exposing the eyes to molecular hydrogen will protect or possibly treat certain eye conditions.

https://pubmed.ncbi.nlm.nih.gov/19834032

https://www.mdpi.com/1424-8247/16/11/1567

But how effective is this approach? Here, I examined early clinical findings, to see what benefits it offers, which eye conditions it might help, and whether those hydrogen "goggles" are more hype than helpful.

How Can Hydrogen Gas Help the Eyes?
Hydrogen gas can reduce oxidative stress — a known contributor to many eye diseases. In addition, studies indicate H2 has **anti-inflammatory effects**, modulating cytokines and immune cell activity, and can **inhibit cell death (apoptosis)** pathways in injured tissues. These combined actions suggest that hydrogen could protect ocular cells (like retinal neurons, corneal cells, etc.) from damage.

There are different ways to deliver hydrogen for therapeutic use. Common methods include inhaling H2 enriched air, drinking hydrogen-rich water, and even bathing tissues in hydrogen water (for example, hydrogen baths).

https://www.nature.com/articles/s41598-020-75492-w

For eye-specific therapy, researchers have tried **hydrogen-loaded eye drops** (saline infused with H2) and **hydrogen-rich water drinking**, as well as systemic inhalation to reach the eyes. The hydrogen goggles being sold fall into the category of **localized hydrogen gas delivery** — they create a sealed environment around the eyes and fill it with H2 gas, somewhat like a mini hyperbaric chamber for the eyeballs. The rationale is that hydrogen gas applied directly to the ocular surface will diffuse into the eye's tissues (cornea, anterior chamber, and even the retina at the back) and exert protective effects.

It's important to note that **molecular hydrogen is very safe** — it doesn't disturb normal physiological ROS signaling and has no known toxic effects at the concentrations used. The main practical concerns with H2 gas are storage and delivery (it's flammable in high concentrations, so it must be handled properly) and ensuring enough gas actually reaches target tissues.

Hydrogen goggles attempt to address delivery by directly bathing the eyes, thus avoiding dilution in the lungs or bloodstream. But does this local delivery actually translate into meaningful benefit? Let's explore what studies have found for hydrogen in various eye conditions.

Hydrogen Therapy in Retinal Diseases

The retina — a thin layer of neural tissue at the back of the eye — is highly susceptible to oxidative stress. Conditions like retinal ischemia (blood flow loss), diabetic retinopathy, macular degeneration, and photoreceptor degeneration involve oxidative damage and inflammation in the retina. A number of studies suggest that hydrogen can be **retinoprotective** in such scenarios.

Retinal Ischemia/Reperfusion Injury:

In a landmark study, Japanese researchers tested H2-infused eye drops in a rat model of acute retinal ischemia-reperfusion injury.

https://pubmed.ncbi.nlm.nih.gov/19834032

This model simulated an acute high eye-pressure attack (like ocular stroke or acute glaucoma) by raising intraocular pressure for an hour. When the retina was later reperfused (blood flow restored), it usually would incur significant oxidative damage (akin to what happens in a stroke). Remarkably, continuous application of hydrogen-saturated saline eye drops during the high-pressure period dramatically protected the retina. Hydrogen rapidly penetrated into the eye — H2 levels in the vitreous (center of eye) rose immediately, and neutralized harmful radicals.

https://pubmed.ncbi.nlm.nih.gov/19834032

Treated rats had *over 70% less thinning of the retina* (a measure of neuron loss) compared to untreated controls. The H2 dosed eyes also showed far fewer **apoptotic (dying) cells** and **oxidative stress markers** in the retina. In short, hydrogen therapy saved a significant portion of retinal cells from dying. The authors concluded that hydrogen eye drops were a highly useful neuroprotective and antioxidative treatment for acute retinal injury, with the added bonus that "H2 has no known toxic effects on the human body". While this was an animal study, it provides proof-of-concept that hydrogen delivered to the eye can protect retinal neurons in extreme oxidative stress conditions.

Retinal Degeneration and Aging:

Oxidative stress is implicated in chronic retinal degenerative diseases like **age-related macular degeneration (AMD)** and inherited retinal dystrophies. Preclinical studies hint that hydrogen might slow such degeneration. For example, a 2022 study found that mice with a hereditary retinal degeneration (rd6 mice) had better photoreceptor survival and structure when given hydrogen-rich water to drink. The molecular hydrogen appeared to have *neuroprotective effects on photoreceptor cells*, the rods and cones of the retina.

https://www.ophthalmologytimes.com/view/arvo-2023-hydrogen-rich-water-in-the-treatment-of-retinal-degeneration

At the cellular level, hydrogen can activate the body's own antioxidant defenses (e.g., boosting enzymes like SOD and GPx) and reduce oxidative damage to retinal cells. In models of **light-induced retinal injury** (excessive light can damage photoreceptors), hydrogen-rich saline has also shown protective effects, likely by quenching the flood of free radicals triggered by intense light exposure.

Emerging research is even testing hydrogen in **human retinal conditions**. A small clinical study in China investigated drinking hydrogen-rich water in patients with *retinitis pigmentosa (RP)*, a progressive degenerative retinal disease. After 4 weeks of consuming H2 infused water twice daily (about 1 liter per day), RP patients showed slight improvements in visual function.

https://pubmed.ncbi.nlm.nih.gov/37860576/

Best-corrected visual acuity improved modestly (on average from ~20/60 to 20/50), and certain electrophysiological responses of the retina (ERG signals) were better than before. There were no significant changes in retinal anatomy over such a short term, but these functional improvements suggest hydrogen might help *slow vision loss* or improve retinal function in RP. The effect was not dramatic — described as a *"slight improvement"* in visual function — but given that RP typically only worsens over time, this hint of stability or improvement from a simple water intervention is intriguing. It's worth noting this was an uncontrolled trial, but it demonstrates feasibility and safety (no adverse effects on eye pressure or general health were seen).

Diabetic Retinopathy and Blood Circulation:

Chronic inflammation and oxidative stress are big factors in diabetic retinal disease. At the 2023 ARVO conference, researchers presented results that hydrogen-rich water may improve retinal blood flow regulation in diabetic mice. In the study, diabetic mice that drank hydrogen water had significantly better retinal blood flow responses to stimuli, indicating healthier neurovascular coupling in the retina. The hydrogen group's retinal vessels responded more normally to flickering light and to oxygen changes, whereas diabetic control mice had impaired responses. Additionally, the diabetes-related overactivation of retinal glial cells (an indicator of stress in the retina) was dampened in hydrogen-treated mice. Interestingly, the hydrogen water group even ended the study with slightly *lower blood glucose levels* than the control group, hinting at systemic metabolic benefits. These findings suggest hydrogen's antioxidant action can preserve retinal function in a diabetes setting — potentially preventing some vascular dysregulation that leads to retinopathy. While this is again an animal result, it adds to the picture that hydrogen interventions might protect the retina from both acute insults and chronic disease processes.

Glaucoma and Optic Nerve:

Glaucoma involves progressive optic nerve damage, often due to elevated eye pressure and resulting oxidative stress in retinal ganglion cells. There is interest in hydrogen as a neuroprotectant for glaucoma as well. We can draw a parallel from the aforementioned high-pressure rat study — it showed hydrogen rescuing retinal neurons from pressure-induced ischemia. In essence, hydrogen acted a bit like a *neuroprotective agent* during an acute glaucoma-like event. Although direct studies in chronic glaucoma models are few, one clinical tidbit comes from Japan, where hydrogen-rich eye drops or water have been explored in glaucoma patients. Hydrogen-rich water has even been used clinically as an adjunct in glaucoma management (one product in Europe, an H2 drink, has been tried for glaucoma). However, an unexpected finding was that drinking a large volume of water, whether hydrogen-rich or plain, can temporarily raise eye pressure in healthy people. This is thought to be due to stomach distension triggering a physiological response affecting eye fluid dynamics. The rise was similar for normal water and H2 water, meaning hydrogen itself wasn't the culprit — just the volume of fluid. The takeaway is that hydrogen supplementation for glaucoma should avoid chugging large volumes rapidly. Overall, while **no miracle cure for glaucoma is on hand**, hydrogen's ability to reduce oxidative injury suggests it could protect optic nerve cells alongside conventional treatments. More targeted research is needed here.

Age-Related Macular Degeneration (AMD):
AMD is driven by cumulative oxidative damage to the retinal pigment epithelium (RPE) and photoreceptors. Laboratory studies have implicated a form of cell death called *ferroptosis* (iron-driven oxidative cell death) in AMD. Notably, hydrogen has been shown to interfere with ferroptosis pathways — for instance, by reducing levels of 4-HNE (a toxic lipid peroxide product) in cells. By lowering such lipid peroxidation, hydrogen might help RPE cells resist oxidative death. This is very early-stage reasoning, but it points to possible benefits of hydrogen for retinal health in aging. Indeed, scientists have speculated that **molecular hydrogen might slow AMD progression** by combating the oxidative imbalance at the heart of the disease. We await clinical evidence, but if nothing else, hydrogen's excellent safety profile means it could be explored as a preventive nutritional supplement for those at risk of macular degeneration.

Figure: Range of eye conditions where molecular hydrogen has shown protective effects in research. Hydrogen's antioxidant, anti-inflammatory, and cell-protective actions have been studied in the **anterior segment** *(dry* *eye, cornea, cataract)* and **posterior segment** *(retina and optic nerve). While most evidence comes from animal models, early clinical studies (e.g. in dry eye and retinitis pigmentosa) hint at benefits.*

Hydrogen for Cornea, Dry Eye, and Lens Health

Not only the retina stands to benefit — hydrogen therapy has been investigated for **ocular surface and anterior segment conditions** too, including dry eye disease, corneal injuries, and cataracts.

Dry Eye Disease (DED):

Dry eye is often accompanied by inflammation and oxidative stress on the cornea and conjunctiva. Researchers have tested hydrogen-based treatments to soothe dry eye. In an animal model of dry eye (induced in rats with a drug causing tear deficiency), treatment with hydrogen-rich saline made a notable difference. Rats received H2-rich saline both by injection and as eye drops frequently throughout the day; this regimen significantly reduced inflammatory changes on the ocular surface. Hydrogen appeared to suppress the NF-κB pathway — a key driver of inflammation — thereby reducing the release of inflammatory cytokines in the dry eye model. Essentially, the hydrogen treatment kept the corneal surface healthier and less inflamed despite the induced dryness. There is also a report of a small **clinical trial of hydrogen** in dry eye patients, in which a specialized hydrogen-generating eye drop or even an H2-producing probiotic was used. The authors noted that hydrogen therapy (even via stimulating gut bacteria to produce H2) showed potential to improve tear stability and symptoms. While detailed human data on dry eye are still limited, these findings support the idea that **hydrogen's anti-inflammatory action can relieve dry eye symptoms**. If you think about hydrogen goggles — flooding the eyes with H2 gas could similarly calm surface inflammation and irritation in dry eye sufferers, although this hasn't been formally tested in a large trial yet.

Corneal Injuries and Surgery:

The cornea, being the eye's exposed window, can suffer oxidative damage from injuries like burns or from surgical trauma. Hydrogen interventions show promise here as well. A study on **corneal alkali burns** (a harsh chemical burn to the eye) demonstrated that hydrogen can accelerate healing. Rats with alkali-burned corneas healed better when given hydrogen-rich saline — the treatment boosted antioxidant defenses (like activating the enzyme Cu/Zn-superoxide dismutase) in the corneal tissue. This suggests hydrogen mitigated oxidative injury in the burn, allowing faster or improved recovery of the cornea.

An even more practical application: **cataract surgery**, which involves ultrasonic emulsification of the lens (phacoemulsification), can cause oxidative stress and damage to the corneal endothelium (the delicate cell layer on the back of the cornea). In Japan, ophthalmic surgeons tried using *hydrogen-rich irrigating solutions* during cataract surgery to protect the cornea. They dissolved H2 gas into the balanced salt solution used to rinse the eye during surgery (reaching about 60% saturation of H2 in the fluid). The results were encouraging: patients who received H2-enriched irrigation had **less corneal cell loss** after surgery compared to those with normal solution. At 1 day, 1 week, and 3 weeks post-op, the hydrogen group showed significantly **higher corneal endothelial cell counts**, indicating fewer cells died from surgical stress (mdpi.com). Clinically, these patients had milder corneal edema (swelling) right after surgery. In essence, hydrogen acted as a shield for the cornea against oxidative insult during cataract removal. This is a real-world clinical use of hydrogen in ophthalmology — and it worked without any safety issues. For someone considering hydrogen goggles, this example shows that **direct exposure of the eye to hydrogen (via liquid or gas) can indeed have protective effects on the cornea** under stress conditions.

Cataract Prevention:
Beyond surgery, could hydrogen help prevent or slow cataracts? Cataracts (clouding of the lens) are known to involve oxidative damage to lens proteins over time. In a classic experiment, scientists induced cataracts in rats using a chemical (selenite) that generates intense oxidative stress in the

lens. When these rats were treated with hydrogen-rich saline injections daily, the development of cataracts was **significantly delayed and less severe** than in untreated rats. The hydrogen likely preserved lens clarity by preventing lipid peroxidation and protein aggregation in the lens fibers. Although this is an animal study, it aligns with the general finding that **H2 can protect against oxidative damage in various tissues**, including the lens. Of course, in humans, the best-proven ways to slow cataracts are UV protection and a good diet, but hydrogen supplementation might emerge as a novel preventive strategy in the future. At least we know it's safe — unlike some antioxidant drugs that had side effects, hydrogen's mild nature makes it an attractive candidate for long-term use.

Do Hydrogen Goggles Work? — Efficacy and Considerations

Given the above research, the idea of wearing goggles that deliver hydrogen gas directly to your eyes starts to sound less far-fetched. The **potential benefits** are there: hydrogen can reach the ocular tissues and might help with conditions ranging from dry eye and corneal stress to retinal ischemia and degeneration. However, we must consider **how much of this potential translates to real-world efficacy** for someone using a hydrogen goggle device at home.

Localized vs. Systemic Delivery:

One advantage of goggles delivering H2 gas to the eyes is that it localizes the treatment. Instead of inhaling hydrogen and hoping enough reaches the eyes via the bloodstream, the goggles bathe the eyes in hydrogen right where it's needed. Hydrogen is a small molecule that will diffuse through the tear film and likely into the anterior chamber (the front interior of the eye) and even further to some extent. In the rat studies, for instance, hydrogen applied to the eye surface was detected deep in the eye within minutes.

So the concept is sound: a steady flow of H2 gas in a closed goggle could maintain a high local concentration, continuously diffusing into the cornea, aqueous humor, and possibly reaching the retina via the vitreous. This could theoretically mimic the protective levels achieved in those successful animal experiments.

Effectiveness and Limitations:

The **effect size** of hydrogen's benefits is a crucial question. The user wisely wonders if the positive effects, while real, might be so small as to have minimal practical impact. It's true that many of hydrogen's demonstrated benefits, especially in chronic conditions, are *modest*. For example, in retinitis pigmentosa patients, the improvement in vision was measurable but not dramatic. In dry eye models, hydrogen reduced inflammatory markers, but it's not as though it cures dry eye overnight. Think of hydrogen therapy as a **gentle assistive therapy** — it reduces oxidative stress and inflammation by a notch, which over time could translate to tissue protection and slower disease progression. It's unlikely to **reverse advanced disease** on its own. So if one expects hydrogen goggles to restore 20/20 vision in someone with macular degeneration, that's unrealistic. But if the goal is to *reduce ongoing damage* or *alleviate some symptoms* (like less dryness, or maybe slightly clearer vision than otherwise would be), hydrogen could indeed have a meaningful adjunctive effect.

Another point: many eye diseases have multifactorial causes. Hydrogen addresses the oxidative/inflammatory aspect, but there might be other pathological processes untouched by H2. For instance, in diabetic retinopathy, there are metabolic and vascular issues; in those cases, hydrogen might help the oxidative stress part, but you'd still need good blood sugar control and possibly other treatments (laser, injections) for full management. **Hydrogen is not a replacement for standard therapies** but could be a supportive therapy.

Comparisons to Other Antioxidants/Treatments:

How does hydrogen compare to existing eye treatments? Antioxidant vitamins (like the AREDS formula for macular degeneration) and other supplements are known to offer some retinal protection. Hydrogen's unique advantage is its ability to easily permeate tissues and selectively neutralize the worst free radicals. It also doesn't risk overdosing – breathing or dissolving hydrogen reaches a saturation point and excess simply leaves the body (often via breath) harmlessly. Traditional antioxidants must be consumed or applied in limited doses to avoid toxicity, whereas hydrogen can be given continuously in moderate concentrations without apparent harm. In acute retinal injury models, hydrogen's benefits (70% preservation of tissue) were quite striking, arguably better than many drugs have achieved in similar tests. That said, for chronic diseases, antioxidants like lutein/zeaxanthin, Vitamin C/E, etc., have proven benefit in large trials (e.g., slowing AMD). In contrast, hydrogen's efficacy in long-term human trials is not yet proven. Hydrogen could potentially complement those supplements – for example, someone might drink hydrogen water and take their eye vitamins too, each working in different ways.

One interesting comparison is with **pharmaceutical anti-inflammatories**: in dry eye, steroid drops or immunosuppressants (like cyclosporine) are used to quell inflammation. Hydrogen would be a far milder approach with likely fewer side effects, but also a less potent immediate effect. It might be more suitable for maintenance or prevention, whereas pharmaceuticals are for active disease flares. In retinal diseases, no antioxidant on its own can match the power of treatments like anti-VEGF injections for stopping blood vessel growth in diabetic retinopathy or wet AMD. Hydrogen isn't targeting those pathways; instead, it may protect cells from oxidative death and thereby complement those treatments.

Current State of Evidence:

It's important to emphasize that *most evidence for hydrogen in eye care comes from animal studies or small pilot trials.* The results are consistently positive in those studies – hydrogen reduces oxidative damage in **cataracts, corneas, retinas, and optic nerves** across various models. Early clinical research (like the RP trial or dry eye experiments) shows *feasibility and hints of benefit*, but larger controlled trials are needed to determine the long-term effectiveness of these treatments. The good news is that hydrogen therapy appears **very safe** and well-tolerated in all these studies, so researchers are pushing forward. According to a 2023 review, H2 therapy has "formally entered the realm of clinical research for ophthalmic diseases," including cataract and dry eye, marking a significant step toward possible medical use. In other words, the scientific community finds it promising enough to test in clinical trials now.

So, **do the hydrogen goggles work?** They are based on sound principles, and if they deliver a sufficient concentration of H2 gas to the eyes, they should confer the same kind of protective effects observed with hydrogen eye drops or hydrogen water. One might expect improvements in metrics like tear stability (for dry eye) or perhaps a slower increase in lens opacity (for cataract) or better retinal function under stress. However, without specific clinical studies on the goggles themselves, we have to extrapolate from the general hydrogen research. It's fair to say that any effect is likely to be **subtle** in the short term — you may not notice a night-and-day difference after a week of use. The benefits of hydrogen therapy could accumulate over time, helping to **preserve eye health and prevent damage** rather than dramatically reverse it overnight.

Where to Find Hydrogen Therapy Goggles

Hydrogen therapy goggles are typically sold alongside the hydrogen generators needed to operate them. The goggles themselves do not produce gas; they rely on an external generator that creates molecular hydrogen, usually through the process of water electrolysis. For that reason, most reputable suppliers offer both the goggles and a compatible generator as part of their product line.

Disclaimer: I have no affiliation with any of the companies that sell these devices, and I do not receive commissions or compensation from their sales.

https://qlifetoday.com/product/hydrogen-goggles/?nab=0

https://www.promolife.com/hydrogen-goggles/

https://hue-light.com/hydrogen-eye-care-goggles/

https://axiomh2.com/product/therapeutic-eye-goggles/

Conclusion

Hydrogen gas is a fascinating new player in the eye care arena. Its ability to neutralize aggressive free radicals and calm inflammation has shown protective effects in a range of eye conditions, from **retinal ischemia** and **diabetic retinopathy** to **dry eye** and **corneal injury**. In animal models and early trials, H2 has helped **retinas stay thicker and healthier after injury,** improved retinal blood flow in diabetic mice, reduced **corneal cell loss** after cataract surgery, and even slightly improved vision in patients with a degenerative retinal disease. These are encouraging signs that hydrogen therapy isn't just snake oil — there is real science behind it.

For consumers considering hydrogen goggles: the device leverages the same concept used successfully in research — delivering H_2 directly to the eye. **Efficiency-wise**, it should work in theory, but individual results will vary. It's best to view it as a *complementary wellness approach* for the eyes, not a standalone cure. Just as drinking hydrogen water daily might confer general health benefits, using hydrogen gas on the eyes could give your ocular tissues an edge in fighting oxidative stress over the long term. If you have a specific eye condition, you should **continue standard treatments** (e.g. glaucoma meds, artificial tears, or retinal specialist injections as prescribed) and possibly use hydrogen therapy as an adjunct if desired. Always discuss with an eye doctor before adding new treatments like this.

In summary, **molecular hydrogen does have genuine protective effects in eye health**, but its impact tends to be moderate. It's not a magic bullet that will immediately fix vision, but it can be a helpful *ally* for your eyes — potentially slowing disease progression and easing oxidative damage in a gentle, safe way. As research progresses, we may see more defined protocols (and proof) for hydrogen in ophthalmology. For now, the excitement is warranted, but tempered with realistic expectations. The hydrogen goggles likely won't hurt — and based on current evidence, they just might provide a small but meaningful boost to your eyes' resilience. Like many health trends, it's an area **"promising but still under study,"** so staying tuned to new clinical trial results in the next couple of years will be key to truly knowing the scope of benefits hydrogen can deliver to our vision.

Chapter 11 - Hydrogen Administration

Incorporating Hydrogen Gas Into a Health Regime

Molecular hydrogen may be supplemented in several forms. Hydrogen gas supplements are popular among athletes seeking to enhance their performance, as molecular hydrogen has been shown to improve endurance and reduce fatigue. Hydrogen gas supplementation is popular among seniors looking to improve chronic conditions associated with aging, Hydrogen therapy is popular for people looking to benefit from its anti-aging properties and to maintain optimum health.

In Japan H2 therapy is used as an approved medical intervention to reduce damage caused by Traumatic Brain Injuries (TBI) and Cardiac arrest.

Daily Dosage

What is a therapeutic dose of hydrogen one must consume daily? The consensus is 1 to 3 milligrams of hydrogen. To figure out how much hydrogen gas you are consuming in H2-infused water, you need to know and understand the gas concentration of the water.

Gas Concentrations

As you investigate hydrogen generator products, you will find manufacturers quote the typical H2 gas concentrations their device can generate or infuse in water. The most common measurements I have come across are Parts Per Million (ppm) and milligrams per liter of water (mg/L)

One ppm of H2 gas infused in 1 liter of water is equivalent to 1 mg/L.

One Part Per Million (1 ppm)

We talk about 1 ppm quite a bit. Let's define this term. One (1) liter of water is equal to 1000 grams. Each gram of water is equal to 1000 milligrams. So, 1 liter of water is equal to one million (1,000,000) milligrams of water. If we infuse 1 milligram (mg) of hydrogen (H2) in 1 million (1,000,000) milligrams of water, the hydrogen concentration is 1 part per million (1 ppm)

Your dosage of H2 depends upon how much H2-infused water you drink. To get a 1 mg dose of hydrogen, you would need to drink a liter of 1 ppm hydrogen-infused water.

This is why companies try to infuse as much H2 into the water as possible, as it will reduce the volume of water you need to drink to obtain a therapeutic dose.

Molar Mass

The molar mass of hydrogen is approximately 1gm/mole. The molar mass of H2 gas is 2gm/mole. I do not use the molar mass of hydrogen or H2 gas to calculate hydrogen concentrations in water.

For the purposes of this book, the ppm concentration is already given in terms of weight per weight. So, 1 ppm H_2 in water is 1 milligram of H_2 per liter of water, (1 liter equals 1,000,000 milligrams)

1 ppm = 1 mg H_2 / L water

However, you may find H2 concentrations reported in:

Moles/Liter) mol/L
Millimoles/Liter mmol/L
Milligrams/Liter mg/L
Parts Per Million ppm
Parts Per Billion ppb

Two common values used are ppm and mg/L. One ppm is equivalent to 1 mg/L.

Gas Saturation

Water is always saturated with gases. A glass of water is saturated with atmospheric gases containing oxygen, approximately 21%, and nitrogen, 78%, along with some trace gases.

Water is considered saturated with hydrogen gas when pure hydrogen gas at one atmospheric pressure (14.7 lb/in) above the water will create a concentration of 1.57mg/L or 1.6 ppm of hydrogen infused in the water. Water ionizers can achieve higher H2 infusion concentrations using pressures above one atmosphere.

Going Flat

Once you generate your Hydrogen-infused water, you want to drink it before H2 gas escapes the water and it goes flat. So, drink the H2-infused water quickly after making it to get the full benefit. Like soda pop, after you open the soda pop, the CO2 gases start to escape from the soda. Eventually, all the CO2 (carbonation) will have escaped and be replaced with normal atmospheric gases. The soda has gone flat. The same thing will happen with an opened container of H2-infused water.

Recommended Dosage:

For water, I have read some writers recommending 1-2 liters and sometimes up to 4 liters per day for athletes. Yikes. I am far more modest and conservative in my consumption of H2-infused water. I top out at 1 liter (1000 ml) or 32 ounces of H2-infused water.

The concentration of H2 gas in my water is approximately 1.5mg/L. By drinking a liter of water, I am ingesting 1.5 mg of H2 gas. According to the recommended dosages of 1-3 mg/H2 daily, I'm on the low side of hydrogen supplementation.

I normally don't drink water, so hydrating with H2 water is beneficial for both water and hydrogen.

Timeframe for Benefits

The time it takes to notice benefits from hydrogen wellness can differ among individuals. Those consuming hydrogen-infused water might observe effects within days to weeks, including better digestion or mood improvements. Inhaling hydrogen gas might show even quicker results, such as reduced muscle soreness or faster recovery post-exercise.

In the long run, hydrogen wellness could lead to improved heart health, better immunity, and anti-aging effects.

"How long does it take to experience the benefits?" When you start drinking molecular hydrogen-infused water, the hydrogen molecules quickly enter your bloodstream and start their work. Some people report a sense of increased energy, mental clarity, improved digestion, and reduced inflammation after just a few days of regular consumption.

Checking Water For H2 Gas Concentration

Gas Chromatography isn't an option for most of us to check H2 gas concentration in water. There are two less expensive alternatives. Although I cannot attest to the accuracy of either method I outline below, I can say that both methods gave similar results regarding the H2 gas concentration in water. For this reason, I will start with the simpler and easier method of using a ORP Hydrogen meter.

Fishawk Digital Hydrogen Meter

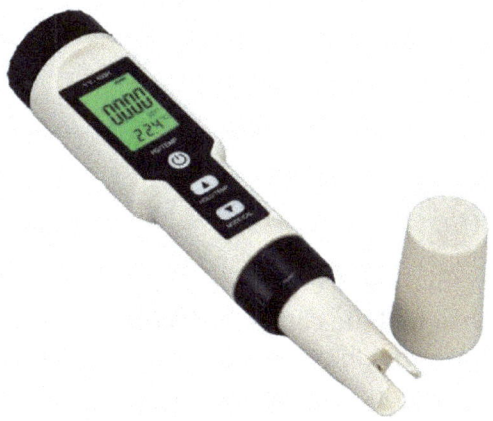

This meter is available on Amazon for less than $20.00 USD. When I tested the device, it provided similar results to the more intensive methylene blue titration method.

Taking measurements couldn't be easier. You place the probe in the H2-infused water and hit the power button.

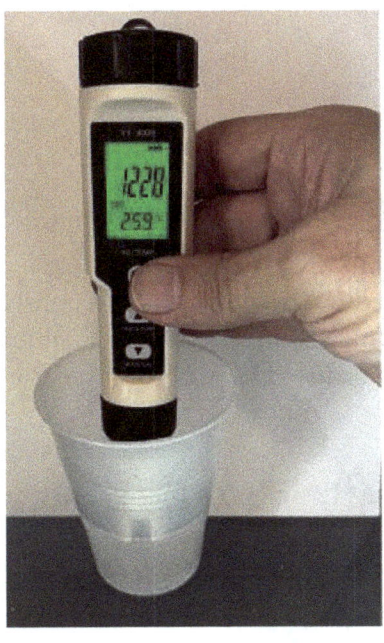
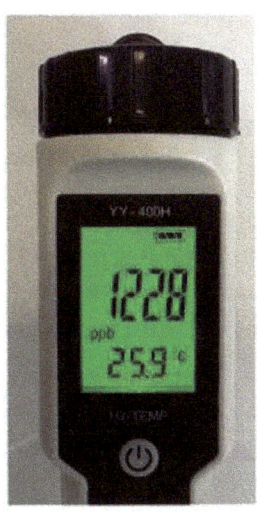

The reading of 1228 ppb converts to ppm by dividing by 1000, which is 1.228 ppm. This is equivalent to 1.23 mg/L of H2.

Amazon

https://www.amazon.com/gp/product/B09YSY2HZZ

Methylene Blue (H2 Blue Test)

Methylene blue, is a thiazine dye often used as a redox indicator in biology and chemistry. Methylene blue can change color in response to the presence of reducing agents; however, it is not specific to hydrogen gas. It has been pressed into service for checking H2 concentration in water.

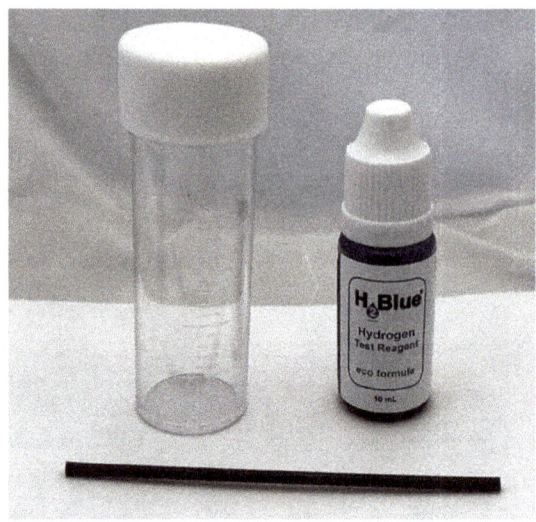

The methylene blue test I purchased was sold as a kit that consisted of a plastic graduated tube with top, a small 10 mL bottle of H2Blue test reagent solution, a stirrer, and an instruction card. The current price is $34.95. See the source below.

H2Blue is a registered trademark of H2 Sciences Inc.

To perform the test, one must fill 6 mL of H2-infused water into the graduated plastic tube. Then add drops of H2 Blue reagent to the water. Gently stir the water until the blue color disappears, then add more drops of reagent until the water doesn't clear. The step-by-step procedure is given below.

The plastic tube is graduated on the side in mL. I found it difficult to fill the tube with the proper amount of water. I found myself either putting a little bit too much or too little water in the tube. Meanwhile, as I am adjusting the water volume, time is ticking away, and hydrogen gas is dissipating out of the water.

To correct this situation, I decided to purchase a 10 mL pipette from Amazon. This made measuring the 6 mL of H2-infused water needed for the test quick and accurate.

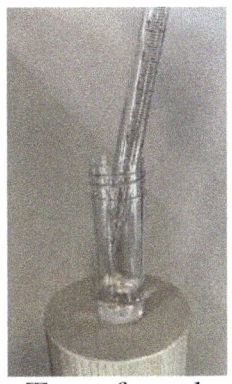 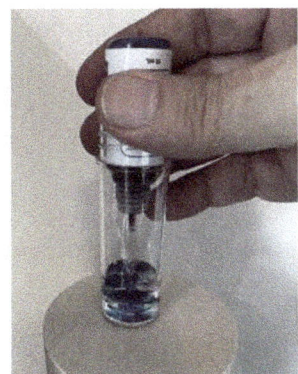 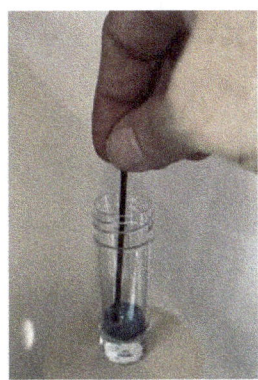

1) To perform the test, place 6 mL of H2-infused water in the plastic tube.
2) Add 5 to 10 drops of the H2 Blue reagent, then gently stir with the provided stirrer.
3) If the water clears in step 2, add 2-3 drops more of the regent and gently stir.

Continue in this manner, adding drops and gently stirring until the water stays blue. Keep count of how many drops of reagent you add to the water.

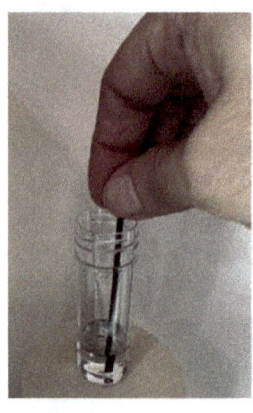 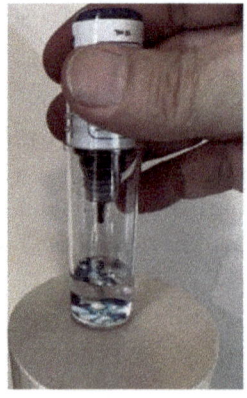 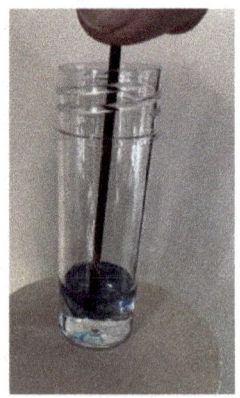

Each drop represents 1/10 of 1 PPM. Therefore, if you add 15 drops before the water turns blue, the H2 concentration is 1.5 PPM

H2 Blue Test

https://h2waterforlife.com/product/h2blue-test-drops/

https://www.amazon.com/H2-Sciences-Inc-Hydrogen-Reagent/dp/B07F6PLCM3

10 mL Pipette

https://www.amazon.com/gp/product/B094D83JZH

Chapter 12 - Hydrogen Generator Products

In this chapter I will examine hydrogen generator products to produce your own hydrogen-infused water.

Hydrogen-Rich Baths and Topical Applications

Hydrogen can also be introduced to the body through hydrogen-rich baths or topicals like hydrogen-infused water. Baths allow for a full-body experience and target specific areas such as joint pain or skin conditions. Some companies sell H2 devices to be placed in large tubs of water, to infuse the water with hydrogen gas.

There are also little misters for H2-infused water for hydrating skin.

H2 Hydrogen Tablets

Effervescent tablets (or powders) that dissolve in water and infuse H2 in the process.

Hydrogen tablets dissolve in water, releasing hydrogen molecules. These are typically magnesium tables that react with water to infuse hydrogen gas in the water. Dr Mercola, who is a trusted name in medical research, sells Molecular Hydrogen tablets. Dr. Mercola states the tablets achieve an 8 ppm (0.0008%) infusion of hydrogen gas in water in an open container. This is an extremely high concentration of hydrogen compared to the concentration of hydrogen under one atmosphere of pressure which is 1.6 ppm.

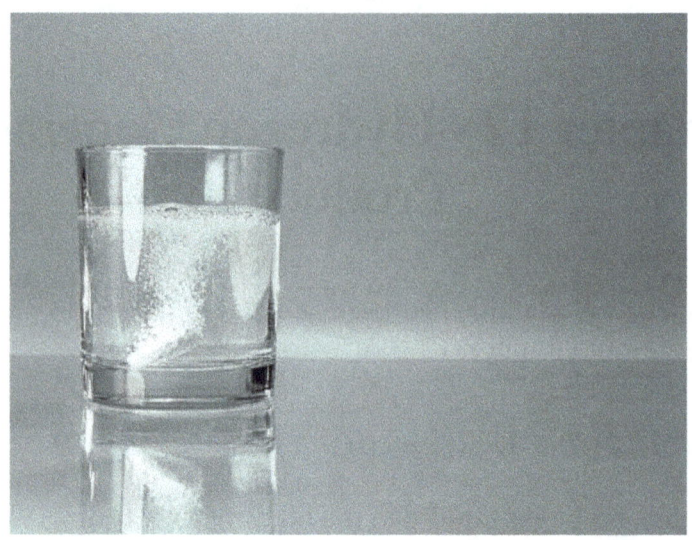

I did not find any lab report on Dr Mercola's website confirming the concentration of H2 gas generated in water from H2 tablets at 8 ppm, and the sales copy for the tablet, reads concentrations "up to" 8 ppm. Achieving such a high concentration of H2 infused in water would typically require 5X atmospheric pressures or about 80 psi. So, how does the magnesium tablet produce such a high concentration of H2 in an open glass? Nanobubbles.

The research I found on hydrogen nanobubbles is exciting but not from what I found is applicable to humans. It is something to keep your eye on as further research is published. And Dr. Mercola may know more than I do about hydrogen nanobubbles.

The added benefit, according to Dr. Mercola, is the residue of magnesium in the water, is essential as a bio-available supplement.

How Hydrogen Tablets Work:

When magnesium reacts with water, magnesium (Mg) and water (H_2O, it effervesces (undergoes a chemical reaction.) This bubbling is the release of hydrogen gas, which then gets dissolved in the water.

$Mg + 2H2O \rightarrow Mg(OH)2 + H2$

I am not a fan of hydrogen tablets, and I don't use them. In addition to Dr. Mercola's product, I know of two other sources for H2 tablets, Allergy Research Group - Molecular H2 Effervescent Hydrogen Tablets and Vital Reaction Molecular Hydrogen Tablets.

H2 Gas Inhalation Machines:

H2 gas can be provided from tanks or electrolysis. Inhalation devices, however, allow for direct absorption of molecular hydrogen through the lungs, delivering its therapeutic benefits to the body quickly and efficiently. This procedure has been used in a number of clinical studies. The treatments can last an hour or more, so it may not be practical for many people.

Medically, H2 inhalation may be the preferred method of administration for quick intervention in the case of Traumatic Brain Injury (TBI), stroke, and heart attacks. People with kidney dysfunction may opt for inhalation because they can not drink enough H2-infused water.

Inhalation machines feed hydrogen gas through nasal cannulas for the user to breathe hydrogen gas directly into the lungs. I am sure they are safe, but for myself, I have the following concerns. First, breathing in too high a concentration of hydrogen gas. This is somewhat circumvented by using nasal cannulas instead of face masks. Second, hydrogen gas is flammable and when mixed with air can be explosive. Third, the H2 gas flow rate of 120-240 mL/min called for in research is significant and challenging to maintain. (However new generation of H2 inhalation equipment easily meets the gas flow standards.) Fourth, adjusting the flow 2-4% rate in the nasal cannulas may be challenging.

To implement H2 inhalation, you need equipment that can safely generate H2 gas at 120-240 mL/min.

One medical study used 2.4% H2 gas mixed with air at 15L/min for 24, 48 and 72 hours. The purpose of the high rate was a medical intervention and to check for adverse effects of H2 administration. The conclusion is that H2 is well tolerated without adverse effects.

https://journals.lww.com/ccejournal/Fulltext/2021/10000/Safety_of_Prolong

ed_Inhalation_of_Hydrogen_Gas_in.11.aspx

Brown's Gas

Electrolysis will break apart water into a gas mixture of 2 parts hydrogen (H2) to one part oxygen (O2). This is called Brown's gas or oxyhydrogen. In electrolysis, there is a negative electrode called the cathode and a positive electrode called the anode. Brown's gas is a breathable mixture of gases, it has a higher oxygen content (33%) than air, with the H2 gas (66%) we are looking to assimilate into our bodies.

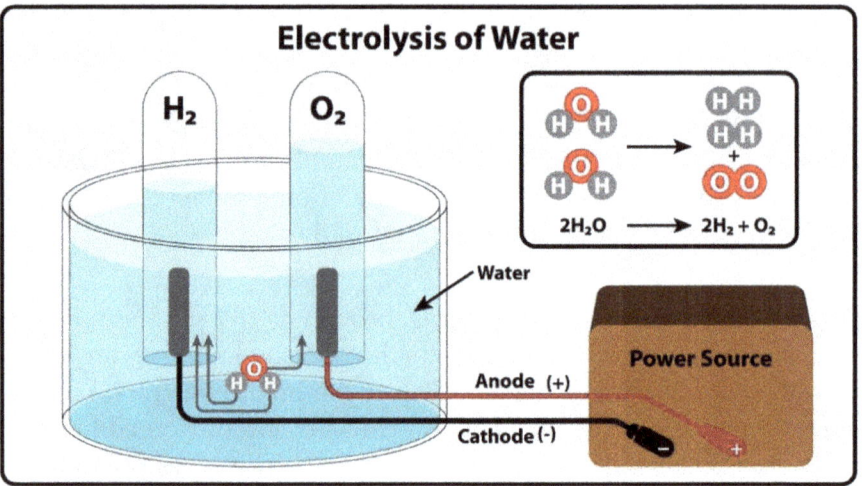

However, Brown's gas is explosive. So, if this gas mixture is allowed to accumulate, you have the potential of a nasty explosion. Think of the Hindenburg!

Brown's Gas for Health: Background, Observations and Medical Data
https://waterjournal.org/current-volume/mohaupt/

Brown's gas generators allow hospitals to implement hydrogen therapy quickly and cost effectively.

A few inhalation H2 generators I have seen for sale are Brown's Gas generators. One unit for sale on Amazon for $2300.00 had a flow rate of 1.5L/min, and does not accumulate generated gas.

Water Ionizers (electrolysis machines)

This is my preferred method of generating H2-infused water.

Quality Matters

When choosing devices, consider quality, reliability, and ease of use. Prioritize items tested and certified for hydrogen content. Device durability and portability are essential factors for those on the move. Lower-quality machines may only achieve 0.5 mg/L or less. Read the product reviews.

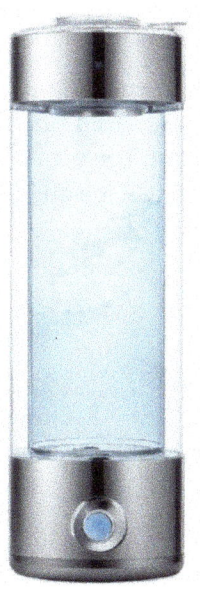
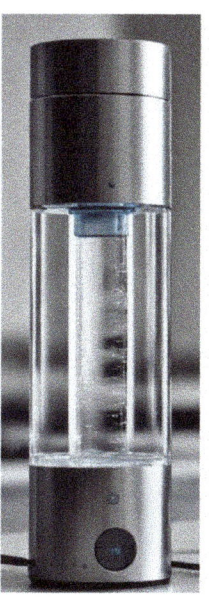
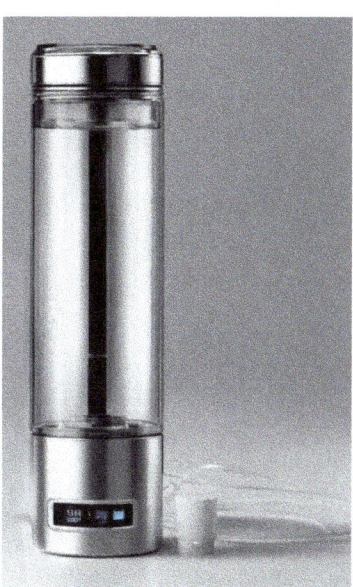

Water ionizers produce hydrogen-infused water through electrolysis. Hydrogen gas is produced at the cathode through reduction, while oxygen gas is produced at the anode through oxidation. Higher quality devices employ a PEM membrane that allows for the clean production of hydrogen gas to infuse the water while venting O2 gas and any chlorine gas.

The gases bubble through the water and saturate (infuse) the water with these gases.

There are a variety of ionizers to choose from. Some have gas adapters for H2 inhalation. However, the flow rate of H2 gas from these devices is too low, in my opinion, to be practical.

Increasing H2 Concentration in Infused Water

Here are a few tips that may increase the H2 gas concentration in your infused water.

1) Fill the ionizer with water to the neck. Only leave a small air gap. This will increase the gas pressure inside the chamber which pushes more H2 gas into the water. Keep the lid tight so no gas can escape.

2) Run the ionizer twice on the same batch of water. Some people will unscrew the top after the first run through to release any H2 pressure. Then screw the top on tight again, and run the water a second time. I tend to run the second batch without releasing any H2 gas. Check with your manufacturer to ensure running a batch of water twice will not cause any damage.

Distilled Water Vs Tap Water

My experience is that tap water will hold more H2 than distilled water. It may be because the tap water has more minerals and makes the water easier to ionize. With distilled water I topped out at 1300 ppb or 1.3mg/L (or 1.3 ppm). When I used tap water, I topped out around 1500 ppb or 1.5mg/L (or 1.5 ppm). This is about a 15% increase in the amount of H2 gas infused in the tap water as compared to the distilled water.

Alkaline Water:

Ionizers that infuse water with Hydrogen may also be called alkaline water generators because the hydrogen-infused water does become alkaline. The oxygen-infused water becomes acidic. However, as we shall see shortly, the O2 is vented, and is not infused into water.

Some people sell alkaline water with the idea that the higher pH levels have health benefits. These waters are typically made using alkali compounds

and not H2 gas. I do not recommend these kinds of alkaline water products for health. I am only suggesting drinking water infused with H2 gas for health benefits.

Gas Inhalation Adapters

Some companies sell H2 gas inhalation adapters for their water ionizers. While a good concept, the, gas flow from the typical ionization chamber made for infusing water with hydrogen, is too low and insufficient to produce the wanted results. Hydrogen gas at 2-4% mixed with air should be maintained at a minimum flow rate of 120 mL/min in a nasal cannula.

Solubility:

Hydrogen gas has poor solubility in water compared to CO2 gas used in soda pop carbonation. Nonetheless, the higher quality machines can produce 1.5 to 2.5 mg/L. This is achieved by bubbling H2 gas through the water. The bubbling gas builds up pressure and helps infuse the water with hydrogen. The pressure created in the home tabletop electrolysis machines is not high and is safe.

Proton Exchange Membrane (PEM)

PEM membranes have been employed in fuel cells turning H2 and O2 in electric power. Now, this type of membranes allows the negative cathode to infuse the water with hydrogen while flushing out oxygen gas through an exhaust vent. Chlorine is added to many municipal water supplies and is a disinfectant to destroy waterborne bacteria. My personal preference is to use distilled water. For this purpose, I own a 1-gallon home water distiller. The added advantage of using distilled water in your H2-Infusion machine is that it will reduce scaling on your PEM membrane.

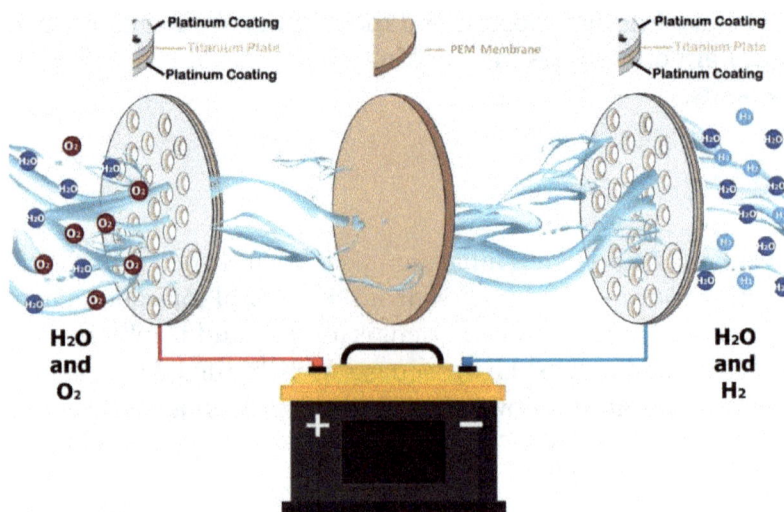

Pros and Cons

Pros - Many H2 infusion ionizers are portable and rechargeable. They can make H2-infused water in a few minutes.

Cons – Cleaning. The electrolysis machines will require proper maintenance and cleaning. Scaling on the PEM can reduce H2 gas production. Cleaning should be performed in accordance with the manufacturer's directions.

PEM Function in Hydrogen Infusion Device

In my device, the PEM is located at the bottom of the ionizer container that holds the water to be infused with H2 gas.

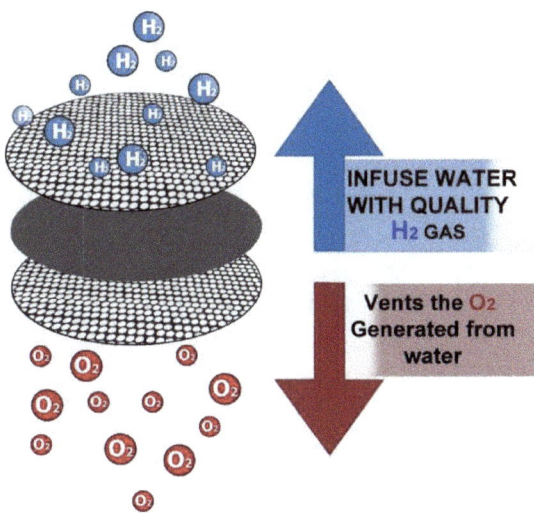

Cleaning Electrolysis-Based Ionizer

These are general instructions for cleaning electrolysis-based ionizers. Detailed cleaning instructions should be obtained from the manufacturer of your equipment. I recommend checking with the manufacturer of your device before cleaning with this procedure.

How often should you clean your device? Depends upon use, but I would recommend once a week.

You can use white vinegar (acetic acid) or FDA food-quality citric acid. Citrus acid crystals may be purchased from Qlife. See the source at the end of this chapter.

Amount of Water - Fill your ionizer midway with hot 100 F water. Pour the water into a cup.

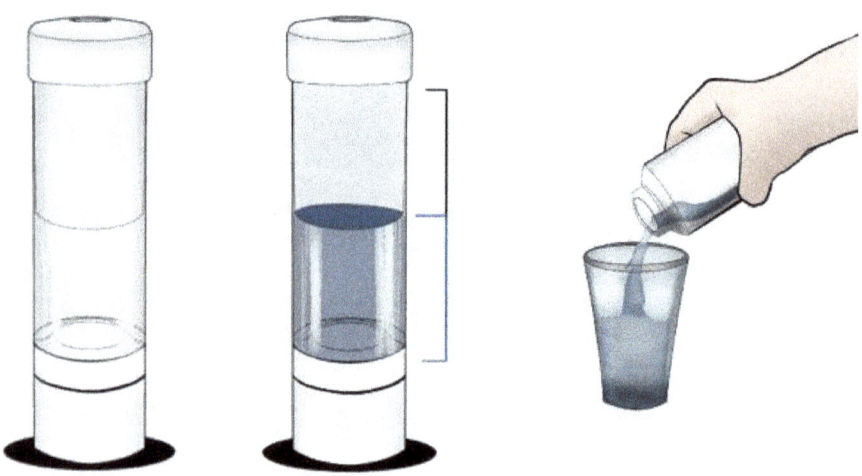

Mix 20 grams of citric acid crystals. This is about four caps full of crystals.

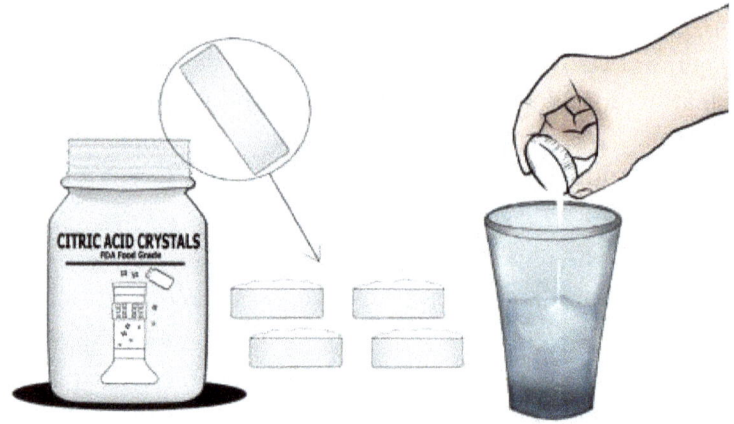

Mix the crystals in the hot water until completely dissolved.

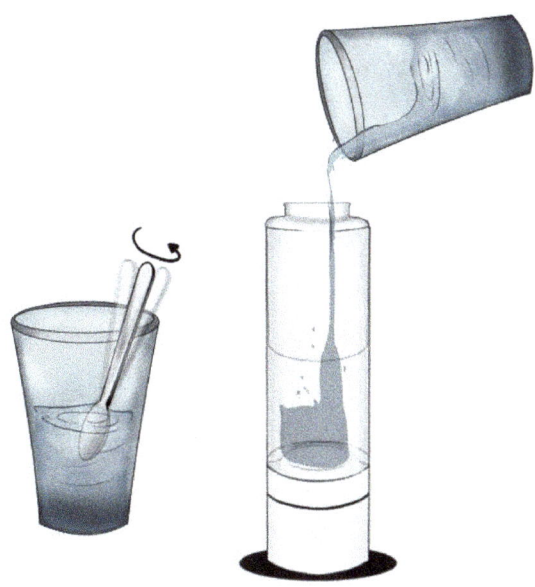

Pour the citric water back into the ionizer. Put the cap on the ionizer and shake the ionizer vigorously for 30 seconds.

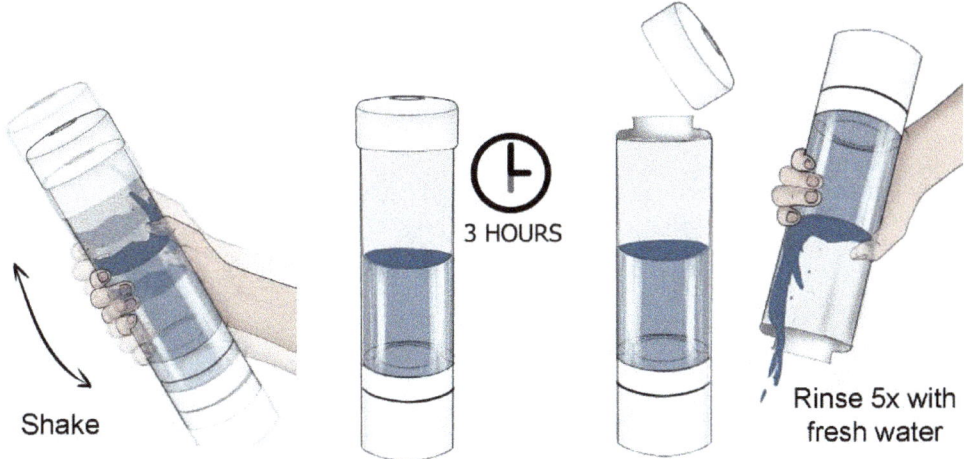

Let the citric acid solution stand in the ionizer for three hours, after the three hours have elapsed, empty the citric water from the ionizer. Flush the ionizer with clean water 4-5 times.

Most PEMs need to remain wet, so after flushing with clean water, leave an inch of clean water in the ionizer to keep the PEM wet. If your device is sitting for a while, dump this water out and replace it with fresh water before using it again.

Source: Citric Crystals

https://qlifetoday.com/product/citric-clean-kit/

Intravenous

I would like to mention intravenous H2 infusion, because it has been used in clinical studies. Saline solutions of hydrogen-infused water injected into the bloodstream have been used in clinical studies with positive results. This is not a typical home method of introducing hydrogen gas into your body.

Chapter 13 – Conclusions

Japan has already approved hydrogen therapy for medical care. It is a safe medical use gas. It is believed that such approval in the United States will be coming shortly.

The first treatment I expect to be approved is in critical care, cardiac or cerebral infarction. Any instance where there is a critical restriction of blood supply, where hydrogen treatment can reduce the damage from oxidative stress.

We have reached the end of the book. If you decide to implement H2 gas in your health regime, please reread chapter 4.

I take a conservative approach to using H2-infused water. I restrain my expectations. There isn't a measured quantitative health improvement to using hydrogen therapy. If hydrogen-infused water provides a 1 to 2 % improvement in my general health over the long run, I'm good with that.

If you are not a water drinker, like me then drinking 16-24 ounces of water per day, hydrogen-infused or not, will at least improve your hydration (and health).

While I would not currently implement H2 inhalation therapy, if I were diagnosed with any neurodegenerative disease, I would plunk down 3.5K and purchase a brown's gas inhalation set-up and start using daily faster than you could say hydrogen.

If you like this book please leave a review on Amazon.
https://www.amazon.com/review/create-review?&asin=B0CN8MPL1R

To send me a comment on this book, use my email address below.
johns-books@proton.me

More Health Books by John Iovine

Benefits of Alpha Lipoic Acid
https://www.amazon.com/dp/B0CH5PHXW1

Red Light Therapy
https://www.amazon.com/dp/B09FC59M4Z

Understanding Fat - The Secrets To Losing Weight
https://www.amazon.com/dp/B09NKDPXPG

Glossary of Key Terms

This glossary provides a concise overview of terms pertinent to hydrogen gas and hydrogen-infused water in the context of health and well-being. Familiarity with these terms aids in navigating the sphere of hydrogen wellness.

1. **Hydrogen Gas**: The universe's smallest and most abundant molecule, molecular hydrogen (H_2), which boasts antioxidant properties and has been researched for its health advantages.
2. **Hydrogen Infused Water**: Water enriched with molecular hydrogen gas. It's an accessible way to introduce molecular hydrogen to the body.
3. **Antioxidant**: Compounds that defend the body from free radicals — unstable molecules known for cellular and DNA damage. Molecular hydrogen is an effective antioxidant.
4. **Oxidative Stress**: An imbalance arising from free radical production and the body's counteraction ability. Hydrogen gas can alleviate oxidative stress, promoting health.
5. **Inflammation**: The immune system's response to harm or infection. Chronic inflammation can lead to health complications, but hydrogen gas has anti-inflammatory attributes.
6. **Mitochondria**: Cell structures responsible for energy generation. Hydrogen can boost mitochondrial efficiency.
7. **Molecular Hydrogen Inhalation**: Inhaling a hydrogen gas mixture for swift absorption and broad distribution in the body.
8. **Hydrogen Water Generator**: Devices employing electrolysis to produce and infuse hydrogen gas into water for home consumption.
9. **Hydrogen Bath**: Soaking in water saturated with hydrogen gas, promotes skin health and relaxation.
10. **Hydrogen Inhalation Machine**: Devices designed for inhaling hydrogen gas, providing controlled delivery for health benefits.
11. **Hydrogen-rich water (HRW)** is water that has been infused with additional molecular hydrogen (H_2), increasing its hydrogen content beyond the normal levels found in regular water.

Understanding these terms enhances comprehension of hydrogen wellness, equipping individuals to make knowledgeable health choices.

Index

Administration, 34
Alzheimer's Disease, 16
Anti-Aging, 26
Antioxidant, 6
Athletes, 23
Baths, 42
Biology, 3
Blood Pressure, 33
Brown's Gas, 45
Caffeine, 32
Cardiovascular Health, 19
Chemotherapy, 33
Chronic Illness, 28
Cognitive Function, 15
Concentration, 34
Concentration Check, 37
Concentration Increase, 47
Diabetes, 28
Digestion, 21
Dosage, 34
Dosage Recommendations, 36
Energy Production, 7
Exercise, 20
Experience, 9
FDA, 14
History of Hydrogen, 1
Hydrogen, 1
Hydrogen Meter, 38
Immune System, 19
Inflammation, 20
Inhalation Machines, 44
Intravenous, 53
Ionizer Function, 49
Ionizers, 45
Macular Degeneration, 19
Medicine, 3
Methylene Blue Test, 39
Metabolic Syndrome, 21
Products, 42
Proton Exchange Membrane, 48
Quality, 46
Red Light Therapy, 11
Recovery, 24
Retinal Degeneration, 31
Rheumatoid Arthritis, 32
Safety, 13
Saturation, 35
Skin Rejuvenation, 31
Sleep, 22
Solubility, 48
Stress, 22
Tablets, 42
Testosterone, 24
Therapy, 5
Time-frame, 36
Vitality, 18
Water Consumption, 14
Water Types, 47
Weight Loss, 30

www.ingramcontent.com/pod-product-compliance
Lightning Source LLC
Chambersburg PA
CBHW071725020426
42333CB00017B/2394